LEAN GENES

A Physician's Guide to Genetic Weight Loss

Eat What You Love, Lose Weight for Good,
and Break Free from Diets and Medications

DR. PHYLLIS POBEE

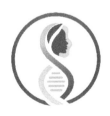

Paperback ISBN: 978-1-0692031-0-6
Harback ISBN: 978-1-0692031-2-0
Ebook ISBN: 978-1-0692031-1-3
Author photo by Brooke Schaal Photography

Published by GeneLean360°

Disclaimer: This book is presented solely for educational and entertainment purposes. The author and publisher are not offering it as legal, accounting, health, or other professional services advice. No income claims are made or inferred in this work. You are solely responsible for your results.

The information provided in this book is not intended as medical advice. While I am a licensed medical professional, the content reflects my personal experiences, research, and opinions and should not be used as a substitute for professional medical advice, diagnosis, or treatment. Readers are advised to consult with their physician or other qualified healthcare providers before making any changes to their diet, exercise, or health regimen. Individual results may vary, and the approaches discussed in this book may not be suitable for everyone. Any reliance on the information provided in this book is solely at your own risk.

While best efforts have been used in preparing this book, the author and publisher make no representations or warranties of any kind and assume no liabilities with respect to the accuracy or completeness of the contents. The author and publisher specifically disclaim any implied warranties of merchantability or fitness for a particular purpose.

The contents of this book are personal opinions and observations based on the author's own experience and should not be taken as anything more than that. Neither the author nor the publisher shall be held liable or responsible to any person or entity with respect to any loss or incidental or consequential damages caused, or alleged to have been caused, directly or indirectly, by the information or programs contained herein. The advice and strategies contained herein may not be suitable for your situation. No one should make any decision without first consulting their own professional and conducting their own research and due diligence. You should seek the services of a competent professional before beginning any program. You are responsible for complying with the laws where you live and where you conduct business. You are solely responsible for the consequences of your use of this material. This book is not intended to diagnose, treat, cure, or prevent any medical condition. Always seek the advice of your physician or other qualified healthcare provider with any questions you may have regarding a medical condition or treatment.

To my mother, with endless love and gratitude: The first person I share all my good news and bad. You have been my lifelong cheerleader, supporting my dream of becoming a physician since I was six years old with unwavering belief in my abilities. When I pivoted to entrepreneurship, your constant encouragement gave me the courage to conquer the unknown and more.

Thank you for being the best Grandmie to my children, my travel partner, my confidante, and the source of so much laughter in my life. Our endless photos and the moments we spend together are treasures I hold dear. You've taught me what it means to dream big, work hard, and always keep family at the heart of everything I do. Your sacrifices, your wisdom, and your love have been the foundation of every success I've achieved. This book is as much a reflection of your influence as it is my journey.

To my beloved husband: I love you beyond words. Thank you for supporting me in more ways than I can count. You have been my partner through every challenge and triumph, walking with me through all the ups and downs I detail in this book.

Without your unwavering belief in me, this book, this company, and this dream wouldn't exist. From the nights you wiped my tears of exhaustion and held me until my self-doubts eroded to the mornings you encouraged me to keep going, you've been my constant source of strength and hope.

Your selflessness, your patience, and your unconditional love have made all the difference. Thank you for being my rock, the strength to every one of my weaknesses, and for constantly reminding me of what's possible when I doubted myself.

Together, we've built more than a life—we've built a legacy. This book is as much yours as it is mine.

To my precious children, with all my love:
You are my greatest joys and my deepest inspiration. At just five
and three years old, you have taught me more about love,
patience, and resilience than I ever imagined. Every laugh, every
hug, and every moment with you reminds me of why I strive to
be my best self. You give me the courage to dream bigger, work
harder, and push through even the toughest days. This book is
for you, a piece of the legacy I hope to leave behind—a reminder
that anything is possible when we believe in ourselves and never
give up. Thank you for filling my world with your boundless
energy, sweet smiles, and endless curiosity. You make every day
brighter and every challenge worthwhile.

CONTENTS

DR. PHYLLIS POBEE

Introduction

You're tired of drowning. Tired of feeling like you want to hide from the world. Convinced you're doomed to fail because you've tried it all but nothing works. I know this because I've been there.

I remember those dark days vividly—days when I didn't want to leave the house because I felt like a fraud. There I was, a family medicine physician, trained to guide others toward health, yet I couldn't even manage my own weight. I felt like I was carrying the heaviness of the world—not just physically, but emotionally, mentally, and spiritually.

Each morning, I'd wake up dreading the day ahead. I'd force myself to put on my white coat, knowing that, underneath it, I was hiding. Hiding from my patients, my colleagues, and, most painfully, from myself. I couldn't bear to look in the mirror because the person staring back at me was a far cry from the confident, capable woman I used to be.

And I really had tried *everything*—every diet, every exercise plan, every so-called "miracle" solution. Each time, I'd start with hope, only to be crushed when the scale barely budged or, worse, when the weight came back with a vengeance. I was exhausted, not just from the physical effort, but from the constant cycle of hope and disappointment. The shame of being a physician who couldn't manage her own health was overwhelming. I was supposed to be the expert, the one with all the answers. Instead, I felt like a failure.

I thought the lowest point had come years earlier, when my brother passed away. The grief had been suffocating then, so I'd turned to food for comfort—only to find that it offered none. But now, a decade later, after I had gone through the worst of the grieving, after I had obtained my medical degree and given birth to two beautiful children, my psyche was just as troubled. I sank deeper into despair, feeling utterly lost and alone. The weight piled on, and with it, the crushing sense of failure and self-loathing. I started to withdraw from life, avoiding social events, avoiding my friends, avoiding anything that might force me to confront the reality of my situation.

If you're reading this, I know you've felt that same crushing burden. You've avoided mirrors, photos, and gatherings because it's easier to hide than to face the reality of where you are. I've experienced this, too. Even my marriage suffered because I felt so disconnected from myself. My energy was drained, my confidence shattered, and my libido nearly nonexistent. I felt like a shell of the woman I once was, and I couldn't see a way out.

And then, as cliché as it sounds, I experienced a lightbulb moment: I couldn't keep living this way—not just for my sake, but for my family, my patients, and my future. I needed something more than just another diet or exercise plan. I needed a fundamental shift in how I approached my health and my life.

That's when I discovered the **power of genetics**. As a physician, I'd always been drawn to science, but even that didn't stop me from trying all the shortcuts—keto, juicing, fasting. Each promised to be the answer, but every time, I ended up back at square one, feeling more defeated. Then I became an expert in genetic testing. For the first time, I saw my body's roadmap laid out before me—a way forward that was finally rooted in *my* biology, not some one-size-fits-all plan. It wasn't another quick fix. It was a breakthrough, a scientific approach that changed how I saw myself and my health forever.

For decades, we've been taught that weight loss is a simple equation—calories in versus calories out. If that were truly the case, wouldn't we all be at our ideal weight by now? The truth is our bodies are far more complex. One-size-fits-all simply doesn't work for everyone.

I realized my struggle wasn't about lack of willpower or discipline. It was about a lack of the right information to understand my body at a deeper level. Once I understood my genetic makeup, everything changed. I started to see real, sustainable results that gave me my life back. Over the next year, I dropped 100 pounds! But more importantly, I gained a new sense of purpose and passion.

This book isn't just about shedding pounds—it's about shedding the limitations that have held you back for too long. It's about reclaiming your life, your confidence, and your future by finally understanding your body's unique blueprint. I know how it feels to be stuck, to feel like you've tried everything and failed. But I'm here to tell you there's a way out, a way forward that's rooted in science and tailored to you.

You may be reading this with skeptical eyes. *Yeah, you're thinking, how is this book going to be any different from the dozens I've read before?* You feel like you've tried it all. But here's the thing: **you haven't tried everything.** At least, not the one thing that finally worked for me and gave me a breakthrough that changed my life in ways I never thought possible.

I created GeneLean360°, a program that combines the power of genetic insights with personalized coaching, nutrition, and fitness plans designed to help women achieve sustainable weight loss and lasting health.

Through this book, you'll learn all about this life-changing program, including these critical lessons:

> ➤ **You think you've tried it all, but you haven't:** Generic diets and one-size-fits-all approaches often fail because they don't consider the unique genetic factors that influence how your body responds to food, exercise, and stress. By understanding your genetic blueprint, you can tailor your weight loss strategy to what works best for you, ensuring lasting results.

> ➤ **You should assess, not guess:** The GeneLean360° Method emphasizes the importance of assessment over guesswork. Through genetic testing and personalized health strategies, you'll uncover the specific factors that have been holding you back and then create a plan that targets your unique needs. This approach not only accelerates your progress, but also helps you avoid the frustration of trial-and-error dieting.

> ➤ **Genetics + Mindset = your path to lasting transformation:** Understanding your unique genetics is the key to finally feeling empowered and ready to achieve sustainable weight loss. With insights into how your body truly operates, you can cultivate a mindset that aligns with your biology, making success feel natural and achievable.

As a physician and a woman who's been on this journey, I am on a mission to share what I learned, so you can take control of your health and live a vibrant life!

Your journey to a healthier, happier life starts here. Through this book, I'll guide you step by step, revealing the secrets that took me from despair to triumph. Together, we'll unlock the powerful connection between your genetics and your potential for lasting weight loss.

This is your moment—don't let it slip away. Let's rewrite your story, starting today.

If you're eager to unlock the deep insights of your unique genetic blueprint, head straight to geneticweightlossbook.com/resources. There, you'll find the options for personalized genetic testing, exclusive tools, and resources that go hand in hand with the strategies in this book. Discover how understanding your genetics can amplify your results and set you on the path to lasting transformation.

DR. PHYLLIS POBEE

PART ONE
THE STRUGGLE

DR. PHYLLIS POBEE

Chapter 1

The Making of a Doctor
And the Weight of the World

I always wanted to be a doctor. It was more than just a childhood dream; it was a calling that resonated deep within me. From a young age, I felt a profound need to heal, to help others in their most vulnerable moments, and to make a meaningful difference in the world. Every evening after high school, I volunteered at the local hospital, my heart racing with a mix of excitement and nervousness. I wasn't just an observer; I was a sponge, soaking in every experience, every bit of knowledge I could.

Even though I was the child of West African immigrants with no other physicians in my family, my resolve only grew stronger as the years passed. When the time came to choose a path for my higher education, there was no doubt in my mind where I was headed. I enrolled in the life sciences program at McMaster University in Hamilton, Ontario—a few hours west of Toronto. Every class, every late-night study session, every exam was a step closer to becoming the doctor I had always envisioned I'd be. The pressure was immense, but it was a pressure I welcomed.

It was during these formative years at McMaster that I met my husband. We were both young, ambitious, and full of optimism. We talked about our dreams late into the night, making plans for the life we would build together—a life where we could balance our demanding careers with a loving family, where we would support each other through the highs and lows of the medical profession.

But as I approached my final year of university, life had other plans. Just as I was preparing to complete my thesis, the culmination of years of hard work and dedication, my world came crashing down. My only brother passed away unexpectedly. The news hit me like a freight train, knocking the breath out of me and leaving me paralyzed with grief. I had never experienced a loss of this magnitude and it was unbearable, a crushing weight that I wasn't prepared to carry.

Grief is a strange thing. It can be all-consuming, a fog that clouds your vision and dulls your senses. In those early days after my brother's death, I felt like I was walking through a nightmare I couldn't wake up from. I tried to focus on my studies, to keep moving forward as I had always done, but it was impossible. Every time I sat down to work on my thesis, my mind would drift back to my brother, and the tears would start to fall.

As if losing my brother wasn't bad enough, just a few months later, I lost my grandfather and grandmother, too. The grief multiplied, layering upon itself until it felt like I was drowning in sorrow. My dreams of medical school were derailed. The path that had once been so clear, so certain, now seemed impossible to navigate. I found myself spiraling into depression, unable to see a way forward.

In my darkest moments, food became my solace. It was the one way I knew to seek comfort when everything else felt unbearable. With every bite, I sank deeper into a hole I couldn't climb out of. I was eating to fill a void that no amount of food could satisfy, and the pounds began to pile on. It wasn't just about the physical weight; I was burdened with emotional weight, too. And not only the understandable grief, but new feelings of guilt and self-loathing, as I became more disconnected from the ambitious woman I once was.

For two years, I put my ambitions on hold, unable to see a way forward. I tried to numb the pain with food and overworking, throwing myself into anything that could distract me from the unbearable emptiness. Nothing worked. I was stuck, trapped in a cycle of emotional eating and self-destruction, unable to find a way out. I felt like I was watching my life from the outside, unrecognizable to myself.

In time, ever so slowly, the overpowering darkness cleared. Eventually, I found the strength to return to my path and go back to medical school. It was supposed to be a fresh start, a chance to reclaim the dreams I had put on hold. But the stress was overwhelming. The rigorous demands of my studies, combined with the lingering grief, led to years of yo-yo dieting. I was constantly chasing after a version of myself that I could never quite catch. One moment, I'd be restricting myself to the point of exhaustion; the next, I'd be eating everything in sight, desperate for comfort.

My body had been through so much, I felt like I was losing a self-inflicted war. I would look in the mirror and see a reflection that didn't match the image I had in my mind. I wanted so desperately to be the strong, confident woman I had once been. Instead, I saw someone who was tired, defeated, and broken.

During this time, I was planning my wedding, and I was determined to lose weight before the big day. For six months, I lived on a diet of liquids, consuming nothing solid for four days out of every week. The weight started to fall off, and I finally felt like I was gaining some control over my life. I lost fifty pounds, but the cost was high. I was weak, irritable, and tearful, barely holding myself together. I looked thin in my wedding dress, but I was far from healthy. My body was screaming for nourishment, and as soon as the wedding was over, it rebelled.

On my honeymoon, the weight came rushing back, and with it, a sense of despair that I couldn't shake. I had done everything I was supposed to do—I had followed the diet, I had lost the weight, but it wasn't enough. The pounds piled back on faster than I could have imagined, and I was left feeling defeated and hopeless. It was as if my body was punishing me for the months of deprivation, for the way I had mistreated it in my quest for thinness.

Then came an ectopic pregnancy. I'll never forget the pain, both physical and emotional, of losing my right fallopian tube. It felt like another piece of me had been ripped away, another dream shattered. The grief pulled me back into that familiar hole of depression, where food once again became my crutch. I was heavier than ever, and I knew in my heart that the combination of my morbid obesity and the loss of my tube was likely the reason for my subsequent infertility.

Desperate to conceive again, my husband and I turned to a fertility clinic. It was a time filled with hope and fear, a rollercoaster of emotions as we clung to the possibility of expanding our family. The clinic visits were a blur of tests, procedures, and waiting. Each step forward was followed by two steps back, and the weight of the uncertainty was almost too much to bear. When I finally became pregnant with my son, I was overjoyed. He was our miracle baby, the answer to so many prayers.

But even the joy of motherhood couldn't pull me out of the darkness completely. You would think the birth of my son would have been cause for celebration, a reason to embrace life fully and come out of hiding. Instead, I found myself retreating further. I was there for him in every way that mattered, except one—I wasn't in the majority of his baby photos. I avoided the camera, ashamed of the way I looked, hiding from the evidence that I had "let myself go." The realization that I wasn't capturing these precious moments hurt me to my core.

I swore that I would lose at least eighty pounds before finding myself pregnant again, but life had other plans. Not long after, I was surprised by the news that I was pregnant with my daughter.

Instead of losing the weight, I found myself gaining even more. The demands of residency, combined with the challenges of raising two young children, left me with little time or energy to focus on my health. I was carrying the weight of the world, and I didn't know how to put it down.

My professional life as a family medicine resident was thriving, but my personal life was unraveling. I was a doctor, a mother, a wife, and yet, I felt like a failure. I was supposed to have it all together, to be the epitome of health and wellness, but I was struggling in ways I couldn't even admit to myself. The pressure to be perfect, to succeed in all areas of my life, was crushing me, and I felt like I was constantly falling short.

One day, after yet another failed attempt at sticking to a diet, I was sitting alone in my car in the parking lot of a fast-food restaurant. The remnants of a meal I didn't even enjoy were scattered on the passenger seat. I looked at the crumpled wrappers, feeling a wave of shame and emptiness. Then my phone buzzed—a photo from my husband. It was a picture of my son holding a drawing he'd made of our family.

He'd drawn himself and his dad in bright, bold colors, both smiling, playing at the park. And in his drawing, I was standing to the side, far from the action, just watching. I hadn't even realized he'd noticed. In his young mind, I wasn't the mom who joined in, who chased him around or played with him on the swings. I was just… there. I felt tears well up, realizing this wasn't the mom I wanted to be.

It would still be another three years before I hit absolute rock-bottom. But this moment sparked something inside of me. If I didn't change, I knew I'd always be on the sidelines, watching life go by. I'd never be the mother, the wife, or the doctor I wanted to be.

I started my journey the only way I knew—through science. I poured myself into everything I'd learned about nutrition, metabolism, and health. Yet even with all my knowledge, it felt like something essential was missing. No matter how many diets I tried or how much I exercised, I kept ending up in the same place, wondering why traditional methods of weight loss just weren't enough for me.

That's when I started paying closer attention to my overweight patients, particularly the women over thirty. I saw their struggles and frustrations mirrored in my own experience. These were women who had tried everything—diets, exercise plans, even weight loss medications—yet they kept finding themselves back in the same place, battling their bodies. And I began to wonder: What if the problem wasn't us? What if these traditional approaches to weight loss weren't working because they weren't designed for bodies like ours?

That simple shift in perspective opened up a new line of thinking. Maybe I wasn't broken—maybe the method I was using to try to "fix" myself was.

Even with this realization, I still felt like I was circling around the answer. I hadn't *quite* landed on it yet. Only three additional years of experimentation, overcoming failed attempts, and moments of doubt unraveled the solution that would change everything.

This is where my real journey began. The path that led me to discover the genetic insights that finally unlocked the answers I'd been searching for. Although I didn't know it at the time, the breakthrough was closer than I ever imagined. Three years later, the turning point came, and I learned the truth about how my body worked at the most fundamental level—through my genetics.

In this book, I shed light on every aspect of this key principle that: **to be successful in losing weight, you must follow a program based on your unique genetic makeup.**

I know how it feels to be lost, to feel like you've tried everything and failed. I know the pain of carrying the physical and emotional weight of that struggle. But I also know there is a way out—a way that is rooted in science, tailored to you, and capable of transforming your life just as it transformed mine.

In the pages that follow, I'm going to take you through the steps that led me to this breakthrough and show you how you can apply the same principles to your own life. This isn't about another quick fix or temporary solution. It's about understanding your body in a way you never have before and using that knowledge to create lasting, sustainable change. Together, we're going to uncover the power of your genetics and use that power to help you become the person you were always meant to be.

No matter how stuck you feel, no matter how many times you've tried and failed, there is a way forward.

And I'm here to walk that path with you.

If this resonates with you—if you feel like you've tried everything and nothing works—I invite you to download a free resource that will teach you the steps toward understanding your own body at a genetic level. Head to geneticweightlossbook.com/resources to unlock the free *Genetic Weight Loss Starter Guide* and discover how your DNA could hold the key to your weight loss breakthrough.

How to Use This Book

This book is here to change the way you think about weight loss—no more quick fixes, no more empty promises. Each chapter is designed to guide you through concepts that challenge everything you thought you knew and reveal the real path to sustainable results. You'll find prompts at the end of each chapter, which you can work through in the accompanying workbook, *Lean Genes Blueprint: Your Transformative Workbook*, which is available for purchase at geneticweightlossbook.com/resources.

Here's what you can expect:

- **Chapters 1-3** will show you *exactly* why everything you've tried so far hasn't worked—and why it never will. From fad diets to relentless cardio, we'll expose why these traditional approaches leave you feeling defeated and more frustrated than ever.

- **Chapters 4-5** dive into why weight loss is so much more complex than "calories in, calories out." Here, we'll examine how grief, stress, trauma, and mindset silently sabotage even your best efforts and keep you from achieving the results you deserve.

- **Chapters 6-7** introduce you to the *game-changer* in your weight-loss strategy: genetics. You'll see how understanding your unique genetic blueprint is the key to unlocking effortless, sustainable weight loss.

- **Chapters 8-20** will help you uncover your *genetic avatar*—your unique genetic profile that influences everything from cravings to metabolism. Each avatar includes real-life transformation stories and step-by-step strategies my patients used to break free from the cycle of failed diets and achieve their goals.

Each chapter includes space for reflections and actions that correspond with the workbook, allowing you to take meaningful steps after every lesson. For those who want to dive even deeper, additional readings are listed in the reference and endnotes section.

Finally, I've provided sample meal plans and workouts toward the end of the book. These are to get you started and can be fully personalized to fit your unique needs. After all, personalization is the key to making weight loss work for you—not the other way around.

■ *Lean Genes Blueprint* Entry: Reflecting on the Weight You Carry

Before starting Chapter 1, let's take a moment to reflect on where you are right now. Purchase your workbook at geneticweightlossbook.com/resources. Begin with this first prompt:

❖ Identify key struggles and emotional moments that have defined your journey with weight.

❖ Define what "release" truly means to you.

❖ Set a powerful intention for moving forward in a way that feels freeing and right for you.

This is the beginning of a journey where you're not just shedding pounds, you're truly releasing what no longer serves you. Let's create space for the best version of yourself.

Head to geneticweightlossbook.com/resources to get your workbook and start reflecting on your journey today.

Chapter 2

One Size Does Not Fit All

Traditional weight-loss methods are nonsense. Too often, they are based on a simple formula of eat less, move more. That sounds logical enough. Which is why so many of us fall for it... Then, we fail. And while, yes, weight loss should be as simple as burning more calories than you consume, if it were that easy, we wouldn't be here.

The truth is many weight loss approaches—whether diets, workouts, medications, or surgeries—often fail because they don't consider the unique complexities of our bodies. These solutions are designed for the masses, based on averages and generalizations, but they don't address our individual needs, challenges, and metabolic profiles.

Why So Many Approaches Do Not Work

Let's take a closer look at why so many of these approaches don't work and what makes them especially challenging for women over thirty.

1. Intermittent fasting: Misguided for women in this age group

Intermittent fasting (IF) promises weight loss by limiting eating windows, but for women over thirty, the hormonal effects of fasting can be counterproductive. Our bodies become especially sensitive to caloric restriction after thirty, and skipping meals can lead to cortisol spikes, making weight loss harder.[1] Fasting can disrupt hormones like estrogen and progesterone, essential for mood, energy, and fat storage.[2] For me, IF caused fatigue, stress, and cravings. Only when I tailored my approach with genetics did I see progress without sacrificing energy or mood.

2. Keto diet: Overhyped and Unsustainable

The keto diet's high-fat, low-carb structure may work for some in the short term, but it's not a universal solution. For women, keto's severe carb restrictions can lead to cravings, mood swings, and muscle loss.[3] Keto can trigger deficiencies if not carefully balanced. When I tried keto, the cravings and fatigue outweighed any temporary results. Genetic insights revealed that my body thrived on moderate carbs, fueling my metabolism and keeping my energy stable.

3. The Blood-Type Diet: Oversimplified Approach

The blood-type diet claims that eating specific foods based on your blood type—A, B, AB, or O—can improve health and promote weight loss. While this idea sounds appealing, scientific research doesn't support it. A comprehensive review in the *American Journal of Clinical Nutrition* found no evidence that following a diet tailored to blood type offers any health benefits.[4]

- **Lacks genetic depth:** Blood type is a minor aspect of your genetic profile. This diet overlooks the complex genetic factors that truly influence how your body processes food.

- **Oversimplifies individual needs:** By grouping everyone into four broad categories, it ignores individual differences in metabolism, age, activity level, and health conditions—crucial factors for effective dietary planning.

- **Risk of nutritional deficiencies:** Restricting entire food groups based on blood type can lead to imbalances. For example, type-O individuals are advised to limit dairy, potentially risking calcium deficiency.

- **Ignores food sensitivities and intolerances:** Food reactions are influenced by various factors like gut health and immune responses, not just blood type. This diet doesn't account for personal allergies or intolerances.

- **Not supported by modern research:** Current nutritional science emphasizes personalized diets based on a comprehensive genetic understanding, lifestyle, and specific health goals—not solely on blood type.

In essence, any blood-type diet oversimplifies the complex relationship between genetics and nutrition. When I delved into genetics-based nutrition, I realized my blood type had little to do with how my body processed food. Focusing on my unique genetic makeup provided a more accurate and effective path to weight loss and overall health.

4. Juicing: Sugar Overload in a Glass

Juicing diets, marketed as "cleanses" to "detox" the body, are often filled with sugar and lack protein or fiber, leading to blood sugar spikes and crashes.[5] For me, juicing left me moody and ravenous. When I pivoted to a balanced approach that matched my genetic needs, I felt stable energy and real, sustainable change without the sugar highs and lows.

5. Calorie-counting: More than just Math

Calorie-counting promises results by limiting intake, but it can lead to starvation mode, where the body conserves energy by slowing metabolism.[6] For me, calorie-counting led to deprivation and binge eating. Genetic testing helped me shift focus to calorie quality over quantity, making calories work for my body rather than against it.

6. Over-exercising: The Trap of "More is Better"

From a young age, I believed that exercise was the solution to weight gain. I started with my mother's step workouts, pushing myself to the brink of exhaustion, and graduated to intense programs like Billy Blanks's kickboxing and P90X. My all-or-nothing approach led to burnout, injuries, and constant frustration when I didn't see results despite my efforts.

For many of us, over-exercising feels like we're taking control, but our bodies may interpret it as stress. High-intensity routines, especially if done without enough rest, can lead to cortisol spikes and even encourage fat storage, particularly around the midsection.[7] This approach also ignores genetic variations in exercise response, recovery, and injury risk.[8] Research shows that certain genetic profiles are more suited to endurance rather than high-impact training.[9]

When I discovered that my genetics favored moderate activity and ample recovery time, I shifted my focus away from intense, daily workouts. I ended up losing 100 pounds without stepping foot in the gym.

7. The HCG Diet: A Dangerous Shortcut

The HCG diet combines extreme calorie restriction with hormone injections. This dangerous mix of hormones and caloric deficits can lead to hormonal imbalances and muscle loss instead of fat loss.[10] Instead of a shortcut, I learned that understanding my body through genetics was the path I needed.

8. Weight-Loss Medications: Quick Fixes with Consequences

Medications like Wegovy, Ozempic, and Phentermine have become popular for their appetite-suppressing effects, especially for women looking for a quick fix. However, they often come with side effects—nausea, fatigue, and gastrointestinal distress.[11] And if stopped, the weight often returns. These medications don't address underlying metabolic issues, stress, or genetic factors that can lead to sustainable weight loss. Instead of relying on an external solution, I found that understanding my body through genetics was the key to lasting results.

9. Weight-Loss Surgeries and Liposuction: Not a long-term solution

Weight-loss surgeries like gastric bypass or lap band procedures can be effective, but they come with risks and major lifestyle adjustments.[12] Similarly, liposuction may remove fat temporarily but doesn't address the root causes of weight gain.[13] Without lifestyle changes, the weight often returns.

Traditional methods create disappointing results. So many of us fail with standard diets, medications, and workouts because they assume we're all the same. Our bodies are unique—shaped by genetics, environment, and experiences. What works for one person might not work for you, and that's okay. It's not a reflection of your willpower or worth; it's a sign that you need a different approach.

Personalized health shifts the focus from generic advice to a plan built around your body's needs. By understanding your genetics, you can make choices aligned with your biology, increasing success and making the process feel natural and sustainable. This is what finally changed my life and helped me lose 100 pounds.

If you're curious about how your genes might play a role in your weight-loss journey, there's an easy way to find out. Visit geneticweightlossbook.com/resources to download a free resource introducing the basics of genetic testing and how it can help you create a personalized weight loss approach.

🔲 *Lean Genes Blueprint* Entry: Reflecting on One Size Does Not Fit All

❖ Reflect on your past experiences with traditional diets, medications, and exercise, and the outcomes.

❖ Consider why these methods didn't work for you and what a personalized approach could look like.

Head to geneticweightlossbook.com/resources to get your workbook and start journaling about your unique path forward.

Chapter 3

The Breaking Point

I remember one specific moment that felt like the final straw. It was during a routine appointment with a long-time patient, a woman in her mid-forties who had been struggling with her weight for as long as I had known her. As she sat across from me, tears welling up in her eyes, she confessed her frustration and shame at not being able to lose weight despite trying every diet and exercise regimen she could find. She looked to me for guidance, for reassurance, and all I could do was nod along, offering the same advice I had given a hundred times before.

But as I listened to her, I realized that I wasn't just hearing her story—I was hearing my own. The words of encouragement I offered felt hollow, empty, because deep down, I knew that I was no different. I was just as lost, just as trapped in a cycle of hope and despair. When she left the office that day, I sat in my chair for what felt like hours, staring at the walls, wondering how I had let it get this far.

The breaking point came later that evening, when I arrived home and found myself standing in front of the refrigerator, staring blankly at the rows of food. I wasn't hungry, not really, but I was searching for something—comfort, escape, relief from the relentless pressure I felt both at work and at home. Without thinking, I reached for a pint of ice cream and started eating straight from the container. Spoonful after spoonful, I felt a temporary numbness wash over me, but it was quickly replaced by a familiar wave of shame.

I pushed the ice cream away, but the damage was already done. I collapsed onto the kitchen floor, tears streaming down my face as the weight of my reality came crashing down on me. I couldn't keep living like this. Something had to change, but I didn't know where to start. The diets, the exercise plans, the countless books and programs—they had all failed me. Or maybe I had failed them. Either way, I was out of options, out of hope.

In that moment of utter despair, something inside me shifted. A quiet, almost imperceptible resolve began to take hold. I knew I couldn't keep going down this path, but I also knew I wasn't ready to give up. I had to find a new way forward, something that went beyond the conventional wisdom, which had let me down time and time again. There had to be an answer, a reason why nothing had worked for me, and I was determined to find it.

That night in my kitchen, after pushing away the ice cream, I knew something had to change. I couldn't keep hiding from my patients, my children, myself. I needed a solution that went beyond yet another diet or exercise plan—something that addressed the root cause of my struggle, not just the symptoms.

In the days that followed, I poured myself into research, determined to uncover answers that had eluded me for so long. I combed through medical journals, attended seminars, and absorbed any science-backed insights I could find. Time and again, the same simplistic advice surfaced: "Eat less, move more." It felt empty, especially after I'd spent years following every diet and exercise plan imaginable with little to show for it.

Then, during one late night of reading, I stumbled upon a field that was on the brink of transforming personalized medicine: genetic testing. It suggested that weight loss wasn't just about calorie math or willpower, but about understanding our unique genetic blueprint—how our bodies were wired to respond to food and exercise. The spark of hope I felt was something I hadn't experienced in years.

This was no quick fix. I didn't just go online and order a genetic test. I dove headfirst into becoming a true expert in the field. As a physician, I knew that simply receiving a report wouldn't provide me with the answers I sought. I needed to understand the science deeply, not only to interpret my own results, but to help others facing the same struggle.

I devoted myself to the study of genetic weight loss, becoming certified in obesity medicine and mastering the complex interplay of genes, diet, and metabolism. I was preparing myself to lead this journey—not just for me, but for the patients who were counting on me to offer something more.

When I took my genetic test, I approached it not only as a patient, but as an expert armed with the knowledge and skills to decode my results and transform my life. The insights were profound. My test revealed a variation in the PPARG gene, which controls fat storage and glucose metabolism, showing that my years of low-carb dieting had been counterproductive. I also learned that my body didn't respond well to intense, prolonged exercise—something I'd forced myself into, thinking more effort would yield more results. With these insights, I tailored a plan that aligned with my genetic profile. It wasn't just a revelation; it was a blueprint grounded in science and refined by my expertise. I adjusted my diet, focusing on actually adding *more* carbs (yum!) and scaling back my exercise regimen to what my body actually needed. For the first time, the transformation felt natural, effortless.

It was then that I realized this was not only my answer, but was the missing link for so many people struggling with their weight. Here's the key: working with someone trained in genetic weight loss, someone who understands the nuances of personalized medicine, is essential. Without this guidance, it's all too easy to misunderstand or misuse the information. This journey taught me that our genes hold invaluable clues, but interpreting them requires expertise— a journey that goes far beyond a simple test and will lead to a sustainable, life-altering transformation.

Here's where I want to be clear: while genetic testing offers powerful insights, it's not something you can navigate on your own. You need expert guidance— someone who can not only interpret the data, but also apply it to your life in a practical, sustainable way. That's why I created GeneLean360°, a program built on my own experience and expertise, designed to help you unlock the power of your genetics without the confusion or overwhelm of trying to do it alone.

This journey of discovery through genetics transformed my life. I realized the same genetic insights that had helped me could help others—especially women who felt like they'd tried everything and failed. This wasn't just about weight loss; it was about reclaiming their health, their confidence, and their future.

That moment on the kitchen floor was my breaking point, but it also marked the beginning of my breakthrough. And now, through this book and the GeneLean360° program, I'm here to share that breakthrough with you.

Self-Assessment Checklist

Answer these questions being completely honest with yourself:

- ☐ Are you frustrated with traditional weight-loss methods?

- ☐ Have you experienced repeated failures despite your best efforts?

- ☐ Are you ready to explore a personalized approach to weight management?

If you answered yes to any of these questions, genetic testing might be a valuable tool in your journey to better health. Head to GeneLean360.com to learn more.

No matter how stuck you feel, no matter how many times you've tried and failed, there is a way forward. Together, we'll unlock the power of your genetics and use that knowledge to help you become the healthiest, happiest version of yourself.

Let's rewrite your story, starting today.

■ *Lean Genes Blueprint* Entry: Reflecting on the Breaking Point

❖ Think about your own breaking points, moments when you knew something had to change.

❖ Consider what you've learned from those moments and what you'd hope to gain from a personalized health approach.

Head to geneticweightlossbook.com/resources to get your workbook and start journaling about your personal journey to breakthrough.

Chapter 4

How Stress and Grief Impact Your Weight

Stress and grief don't just weigh on the mind—they reshape the body. They change our hormones, disrupt metabolism, and alter the way we process food and energy. I learned this firsthand as I navigated some of the most painful moments of my life, unaware that my body wasn't betraying me—it was trying to protect me.

For years, I was trapped in an exhausting cycle—stress, emotional eating, guilt, repeat. I thought my struggles were a matter of willpower, but what I didn't realize was that stress and grief weren't just emotional experiences—they were triggering physiological responses that directly impacted my metabolism, hormones, and weight.

It wasn't until years later—after my desperate attempts to lose weight for my wedding, the devastation of an ectopic pregnancy, and finally having my two children—that I turned to genetic testing and uncovered something life-changing: my body wasn't broken. It was responding exactly the way it was wired to under stress. And more importantly, I learned how to work *with* my biology instead of feeling like I was constantly fighting against it.

But my struggles with emotional eating didn't begin with my wedding or my fertility journey. They started nearly a decade earlier, with a loss that changed everything.

The Loss of My Brother: The Beginning of Emotional Eating

The sudden loss of my brother was one of the most devastating experiences of my life. At the time, I had no idea how much it would shape my relationship with food for years to come. In the depths of grief, I turned to food for comfort, searching for relief from an ache that felt unbearable.

But the more I ate, the more the weight piled on—and with it came an unbearable sense of guilt and shame. I tried to restrict myself, forcing my way into diets that felt like punishment. But no matter how hard I fought to regain control, my body fought back.

At the time, I didn't realize that my cravings, weight gain, and exhaustion weren't signs of weakness—they were signs of a body in survival mode. The stress of losing my brother triggered a surge in cortisol, the body's primary stress hormone, designed to protect us during prolonged stress. But instead of helping, this biological response was working against me—driving up cravings, slowing my metabolism, and making weight loss feel impossible.

And I know I'm not alone in this.

Maybe your story didn't begin with the loss of a loved one. Maybe for you, it was a breakup that left you feeling like you weren't enough. Or a health scare that made you see your body as something to fear. Maybe it was the weight of always trying to measure up, never quite feeling like you belonged. Or perhaps it was something quieter—years of chronic stress, each day adding a little more pressure until suddenly, one day, you looked in the mirror and didn't recognize yourself.

Whatever it was, I bet you can pinpoint the moment you first felt like you were losing yourself. The moment when food, or another coping mechanism, became a way to dull the pain, fill the void, or regain a sense of comfort—even if only for a little while.

Recognizing where it all began is one of the most powerful steps toward understanding how stress, grief, and even seemingly small emotional wounds impact not just your mind, but your entire physical being.

The good news? You can break free. You can reconnect with your body and reshape your journey in a way that aligns with your biology, your needs, and your future. And as we explore my own journey through stress and grief, I hope you'll begin to see your own struggles in a new light.

The Stress of Infertility: A Vicious Cycle

By the time my wedding approached, I was no stranger to using food to cope with stress. But this time, I took it to the extreme—liquid diets, deprivation, and punishing workouts. And after my honeymoon, when the weight I had lost came rushing back, I was on an emotional rollercoaster.

The physical pain of my ectopic pregnancy was intense—but the emotional toll? Unbearable. I was already trying to heal, trying to rebuild my trust in my body—only to be met with another devastating blow. Infertility wasn't just a medical condition; it was a relentless emotional war. Every single month, hope rose—only to be crushed again. Every negative test, every failed attempt, was another silent heartbreak, deepening the belief that my body had betrayed me.

I was caught in a vicious loop—the stress of infertility fueled weight gain, and that weight gain seemed to deepen my infertility. The more I obsessed over losing weight, the more my body resisted. And the guilt of knowing this only fed the cycle, making me feel trapped in a body I no longer trusted.

Chronic stress elevates cortisol levels, which signals the body to store fat—especially in the abdomen—because it perceives prolonged stress as a sign of famine or danger. This hormonal shift not only makes weight loss harder, but also disrupts reproductive hormones, making conception even more difficult.

Perhaps you've felt the frustration of doing everything right—following the diets, pushing through the workouts— only to see little to no progress. Or maybe you, like me, have spent years believing that if you could just muster enough discipline, you could finally take control of your body.

But the truth I had to learn was this: You don't heal by punishing yourself. The more we fight against our bodies, the more they fight back. Our biology isn't the enemy—it's trying to protect us. And once I truly understood how deeply stress was affecting my body, I was finally able to break free from the cycle.

The Weight of Grief and Healing from Loss

Losing a pregnancy is more than just a physical loss—it's the loss of a future you had already begun to imagine. What I didn't realize at the time was that grief itself changes the body. Chronic stress and emotional pain trigger the release of cortisol, a hormone that increases appetite and promotes fat storage—especially around the abdomen. Grief often leads to depression, which can drain motivation, disrupt hunger signals, and create a disconnect between what we know we should do and what we feel capable of doing.

If you're in that place now—grieving, struggling, feeling trapped in your own body—I want you to know that there is a way forward. Healing doesn't come from restriction or self-blame. It comes from learning how to support your body through the storm, not fight against it.

A Turning Point: Finding a New Path

Holding my miracle son in my arms should have been the moment of complete healing—but instead, I was still carrying the weight, both physically and emotionally, of everything I had endured. I avoided photos, hiding from the evidence of what I perceived as failure, and promised myself I would lose weight before having another child.

When my second pregnancy surprised me before I had begun to heal, I found myself spiraling deeper. Between residency demands and raising young children, I was overwhelmed and still caught in the same destructive patterns.

For years after, I battled the same cycles of stress, emotional eating, and failed diets. I tried every plan imaginable, but nothing worked—because I was still treating the symptoms, not the root cause.

It wasn't until I turned to genetic testing that everything changed. For the first time, I understood my body on a genetic level. I discovered how my body uniquely responded to food, exercise, and stress, and I learned that my struggles weren't about willpower at all—they were about biology. Once I started working with my body instead of against it, the weight began to come off, and the mental and emotional fog lifted.

This was the moment everything changed. For years, I thought my body was the problem—until I realized it was the key to the solution all along. And this could be your turning point, too. Imagine no longer guessing or blaming yourself, but instead having real answers—answers that finally make sense of your body, your metabolism, and your struggles.

The path forward isn't about restriction or shame. It's about understanding. And once you truly understand your body, everything changes.

Breaking the Cycle of Emotional Eating

Understanding how my genetics influenced my body's response to stress helped me unlock another critical piece of my struggle—emotional eating. For years, this pattern had controlled me. I turned to food for comfort, to numb the grief, the stress, and the weight of feeling like I had failed my body. But as I began to understand my genetics, everything changed. Instead of using food as an emotional crutch, I learned how to fuel my body in a way that nourished and supported it.

Through genetic testing, I discovered that my body was wired to hold onto weight under stress. My metabolism wasn't broken—it was responding to my hormonal environment. Grief, anxiety, and chronic stress had triggered biological processes that made weight loss feel impossible. Once I understood this, I stopped blaming myself. My past struggles weren't about willpower or discipline; they were about working against my own biology.

With this new awareness, I shifted my focus to healing from the inside out. I learned how to eat in a way that worked *with* my genetic blueprint rather than against it. For me, this meant prioritizing protein at breakfast to balance my blood sugar, incorporating specific anti-inflammatory foods that worked with my genetic profile, and timing my meals to optimize my natural metabolic rhythms. And as I made these personalized changes, something incredible happened: the weight began to come off—not through restriction or punishment, but through alignment. My energy increased. My mind felt clearer. The emotional fog that had weighed me down for years finally started to lift.

If emotional eating has been a struggle for you, know that you're not alone—and more importantly, that you *can* break free. Here are some practical steps to begin reclaiming control:

1. **Identify Your Emotional Triggers.** Pay attention to what drives your eating patterns. Is it stress? Anxiety? Grief? Self-doubt? Emotional eating isn't just about food—it's about how we cope with emotions. Recognizing these triggers is the first step toward healing.

2. **Understand Your Body's Stress Response.** If you've struggled with weight gain under stress, it's not just in your head—it's in your biology. Chronic stress elevates cortisol, which increases appetite and promotes fat storage. Learning how *your* body uniquely responds to stress can help you create a strategy that works for you, not against you.

3. **Reframe Your Relationship with Food.** Food isn't the enemy, and neither is your body. Instead of restrictive dieting, focus on nourishment. Ask yourself, *Is this fueling my body, or is this feeding my emotions?* That simple question can shift the way you approach eating.

4. **Implement Stress-Management Techniques.** Based on your genetic makeup, certain stress-relief methods may work better for you than others. For some, it might be gentle movement like yoga or walking; for others, it might be meditation or deep breathing exercises. Finding what works for your body's unique stress response can dramatically impact your eating patterns.

5. **Seek Professional Support.** Healing isn't meant to be done alone. Whether it's working with a therapist, coach, or health professional, seeking guidance can help you address the deeper emotions behind emotional eating and create a sustainable path forward.

6. **Give Yourself Grace.** Breaking free from emotional eating isn't about perfection—it's about progress. Every step you take toward understanding and honoring your body is a victory.

The moment I stopped seeing my body as the problem and started working with it instead of against it, everything changed. And when you discover your own genetic blueprint and learn to work with your biology rather than fighting against it, your relationship with food and your body can transform in ways you never thought possible.

Free Resources to Support Your Journey

To help you apply the strategies we've discussed for managing stress and breaking free from emotional eating, I've created a set of free resources to guide and support you on your path to working *with* your unique genetic blueprint.

For more detailed information and practical tools, visit **geneticweightlossbook.com/resources** to download the following:

- **Stress Management Techniques** – Discover effective ways to regulate stress and calm your nervous system, including deep-breathing exercises, progressive muscle relaxation, and mindfulness meditation.

- **The Role of Cortisol in Weight Gain** – Learn how elevated cortisol levels impact metabolism, fat storage, and cravings—and explore evidence-based strategies to bring your stress hormones back into balance through sleep, movement, and nutrition.

- **Healthy Coping Strategies for Stress and Grief** – Find supportive alternatives to emotional eating, such as engaging in fulfilling hobbies, strengthening social connections, and developing personalized self-care routines.

Lean Genes Blueprint Entry: Reflecting on How Stress and Grief Impact Your Weight

- ❖ Identify emotional triggers—stress, grief, guilt— that may be affecting your metabolism and eating patterns.

❖ Recognize how these emotions shape your behaviors and weight struggles.

❖ Develop personalized strategies to create a healthier relationship with food and break free from unhealthy cycles.

Head to geneticweightlossbook.com/resources to get your workbook and start journaling about how stress and grief have shaped your health journey

This is your opportunity to gain clarity, reconnect with your body, and take the first step toward lasting transformation.

Remember, your body isn't broken—it's responding exactly as it was designed to under stress. The key is understanding your unique genetic blueprint and learning to work with it, not against it. Once you stop fighting your biology and start working with it, everything changes.

DR. PHYLLIS POBEE

PART TWO

THE SOLUTION

DR. PHYLLIS POBEE

Chapter 5

The Power of Mindset

For years, I thought that weight loss was all about willpower. If I could just push myself harder, follow the diet perfectly, or stay consistent with exercise, the results would come. As I cycled through one failed diet after another, it became clear that something was missing in this mindset. It wasn't about trying harder. It was about understanding myself and my body in a new way.

When I discovered genetic testing, everything changed. Suddenly, I could let go of the idea of willpower and work with my body's unique blueprint. This shift from frustration to empowerment was rooted in a fundamental mindset change, one that has shaped my journey and allowed me to regain my health, confidence, and energy.

From Shame to Understanding

As I shared in the earlier chapters, my life was filled with stress—first as a student, then as a grieving sister, and later as a mother of two toddlers. Every stressful event seemed to pile onto the last, and the emotional toll it took on me manifested in my weight. Instead of acknowledging the impact of these life events, I blamed myself for every pound I gained.

I'd cycle through diets like a revolving door, each one promising to be "the one" that would finally work. Yet every failed attempt left me feeling more defeated, more ashamed, and more convinced I was destined to live in this prison of my own making. I withdrew from social events, canceled plans, and avoided friends because the thought of being seen—and being judged—was unbearable.

It wasn't just about my weight anymore. My confidence eroded to the point where even the smallest tasks felt insurmountable. The worst part was that I started to believe that this was just my life—that I was stuck.

Vulnerability and Community

Then something unexpected happened. I began to share my story. I told people about my years of unsuccessful dieting and how each failure left me feeling more and more hopeless. What happened next was remarkable: women— friends, colleagues, even patients—started opening up to me about their own struggles. It was as if my vulnerability gave them permission to be honest about their battles with weight, health, and self-esteem.

I wasn't alone in this. There were so many others just like me, who felt trapped in a cycle of frustration and failure, all because they were chasing solutions that didn't address their unique needs.

These conversations didn't just launch me into the world of weight loss and genetics—they also helped me realize how much our mindset shapes our outcomes. Many of the women I spoke to were stuck in a cycle of negative self-talk, convinced they weren't worthy of success or happiness. They sabotaged their own progress because, deep down, they didn't believe change was possible.

Change Your Mind, Change Your Life

This is where the real work began. *Changing your mind is the first step in changing your life.* Before I could change my body, I had to change the way I thought about myself, my health, and my relationship with food and exercise. I had to let go of the guilt and shame that had been holding me back, and I had to replace it with a sense of empowerment and self-compassion.

One of the most powerful lessons I learned was that *my struggles with weight weren't my fault.* I had been doing the best I could with the information I had. But now, armed with new information about my genetics, I could make better choices and work in alignment with my body, not against it.

This shift in mindset was crucial. It allowed me to stop viewing my weight loss journey as a series of failures and start seeing it as an opportunity to learn, grow, and evolve. *Mindset became the foundation on which everything else was built.* Without it, I would have continued to sabotage myself, fall back into old patterns, and give up at the first sign of struggle.

The Power of Personalized Knowledge

The catalyst for my transformation wasn't just mindset, of course. As I have said, the key was genetic testing. With the insights from my genetic blueprint, I learned how my body responds to certain foods, exercises, and even stress. Suddenly, I wasn't battling an invisible enemy anymore; I was equipped with the knowledge I needed to make informed choices.

For the first time, I could tailor my diet and exercise routine based on what I *knew* would work for my body, not just what worked for someone else. This new level of personalization empowered me to reframe my approach to health, and the weight started to come off. More than that, though, *I started to feel like myself again*—stronger, more confident, and more in tune with my body than I had been in years.

Actionable Steps to Reprogram Your Mindset

Your genetics are the missing piece to effortless weight loss. They reveal why some diets fail, why cravings persist, and why your body reacts the way it does. When you combine this knowledge with the right mindset, you unlock the power to work with your body, not against it.

These five steps will show you how to shift your thoughts, align with your genetic strengths, and create lasting transformation.

1. **Acknowledge the role of mindset:** Your mindset is more powerful than any diet or workout plan. Start by recognizing how your thoughts might be holding you back from achieving lasting success.

2. **Get your genetic blueprint:** Like I did, you need to understand your body at a deeper level. Get a genetic test consultation by visiting GeneLean360.com and learn how your unique genetic makeup influences your metabolism, cravings, and response to exercise.

3. **Shift from blame to empowerment:** Stop blaming yourself for past failures. Understand that weight

loss isn't a one-size-fits-all solution, and your struggles don't define you.

4. **Celebrate progress, not perfection:** Focus on the small wins—each step forward is progress. Don't let perfectionism hold you back from celebrating how far you've already come.

5. **Cultivate self-compassion:** Be kind to yourself on this journey. Weight gain during times of stress or grief is not a failure; it's a biological response. Self-compassion will keep you moving forward, even when times get tough.

Embrace the Journey with Confidence

As I began to see my body change, I realized that the true transformation wasn't just about losing weight—it was about gaining control over my mindset and my life. I had the tools I needed, and I wasn't fighting against myself anymore.

You have that same power. As you continue this journey, I encourage you to reflect on your own mindset.

❖ What beliefs are holding you back?

❖ What would it feel like to let those go?

Remember, this isn't just about shedding pounds—it's about reclaiming your confidence and your sense of self-worth. You are capable. You are worthy. And with the right tools and mindset, you can achieve the transformation you've been longing for.

You can always find support at GeneLean360.com. When you visit our website, you can access a genetic testing consultation where you'll get a personalized weight loss plan.

▣ *Lean Genes Blueprint* Entry: Reflecting on The Power of Mindset

- ❖ Identify any beliefs or thoughts that might be holding you back on your health journey.

- ❖ Explore how shifting your mindset could open the door to a more fulfilling path forward.

Have you ordered your Lean Genes Blueprint workbook yet? Now's the time to commit to taking action! Head to geneticweightlossbook.com/resources to grab it.

Chapter 6

Genetics 101

Mindset is the key that unlocks the door to transformation. However, once that door is open, it's time to step through and take action. For me, the first real action step was to understand my genetics—not just as a concept, but as a guide to every decision I would make from that point forward.

Genetics is the foundation of personalized health. When it comes to weight loss, it's a game-changer. By analyzing the specific genes linked to metabolism, fat storage, appetite, and even food preferences, we can gain a deeper understanding of why our bodies respond the way they do. This knowledge allows us to tailor our lifestyle choices in a way that aligns with our genetic predispositions, making it easier to achieve and maintain our health goals.

What Genetic Testing Tells Us

So, you may be wondering: what exactly *is* genetic testing, and how does it work? Genetic testing for weight loss is a non-invasive process that usually involves a simple saliva or cheek swab sample, making it quick and painless. This sample is then sent to a lab, where specialized testing is performed to analyze specific genes associated with metabolism, fat storage, and other health factors that influence weight. Rather than examining your entire genome, genetic testing for weight loss zooms in on specific genetic markers, known as SNPs (single nucleotide polymorphisms).

SNPs are small variations in DNA that can have a significant impact on how your body functions. These tiny differences help determine traits like how your body responds to carbohydrates, your predisposition for storing fat, and even how well you handle certain types of exercise. By analyzing SNPs linked to weight and metabolism, genetic testing provides insights that go beyond general advice, giving you a precise understanding of what's most relevant to *your* unique biology.

Here are some of the key areas that genetic testing can illuminate:

Metabolism: Certain SNPs affect how efficiently your body burns calories. Some people are genetically predisposed to a faster metabolism, while others may have a slower one. Understanding your metabolic rate can help you adjust your caloric intake and exercise routine to better match your body's natural tendencies.

Fat storage: Some SNPs influence where and how your body stores fat. For instance, certain genetic markers are linked to a higher likelihood of storing fat in the abdominal area, which is associated with increased health risks. Knowing this can guide you in targeting specific areas through tailored exercise and nutrition strategies.

Carbohydrate and fat sensitivity: SNPs can also affect how your body processes different macronutrients. For example, some people are more sensitive to carbohydrates, leading to blood-sugar spikes and increased fat storage, while others may be more efficient at metabolizing fats. This insight can help you determine the right balance of carbs, fats, and proteins in your diet.

Appetite and satiety: Have you ever wondered why some people feel full after a small meal while others need more to feel satisfied? SNPs play a role in regulating hunger hormones, such as ghrelin and leptin, which influence your appetite and satiety. Understanding your genetic predisposition can help you manage hunger and avoid overeating.

Exercise response: Not all exercise is equally effective for everyone. Some SNPs indicate a genetic predisposition for excelling at endurance-based activities, while others suggest a stronger response to strength training or high-intensity interval training (HIIT). By understanding your genetic response to exercise, you can create a workout plan that maximizes your results and keeps you motivated.

Genetic testing, through the analysis of SNPs, provides a powerful lens into these areas, allowing you to personalize your health approach based on scientific insights unique to you. This knowledge is both empowering and transformative, enabling you to make decisions that align with your body's natural inclinations and pave the way to sustainable results.

The struggle you've experienced with weight loss is not just in your head; it's in your genes. The simplistic "calories in, calories out" view fails to account for the complex interplay between our genetics and our environment. Your genes influence how your body metabolizes food, how it stores fat, how it responds to exercise, and even how it regulates hunger and satiety.[14]

The Science of Genetic Influence on Weight research shows that up to seventy percent of the variance in body weight can be attributed to genetic factors.[15] This means that while diet and exercise are important, they are only part of the equation. Understanding the genetic factors at play in your body can help you create a personalized strategy that works for you.

Several key genes that influence weight management have been identified. For example, the FTO gene (fat mass and obesity-associated gene), which has been widely studied.[16] Variations in this gene can predispose individuals to store excess calories as fat, particularly in response to a diet high in refined carbohydrates and sugars.[17] Another important gene is the MC4R **gene**, which plays a critical role in regulating appetite. Variants of this gene can make it harder to feel full after eating, leading to increased food intake and weight gain.[18]

These genetic markers are crucial to understanding why traditional weight-loss methods may not have worked for you. For example, if you have a genetic predisposition to insulin resistance, you might struggle with diets that are high in carbohydrates, even if they are otherwise "healthy."[19] Similarly, if your body doesn't metabolize fats efficiently, a high-fat, low-carb diet might not be the best approach for you.[20]

Given the significant role that genetics play in weight management, it becomes clear that a one-size-fits-all approach to weight loss is not only ineffective, it is also counterproductive.[21] Each person's genetic makeup is unique, which means that the most effective weight loss strategies must be personalized.

By recognizing the limitations of traditional approaches and embracing a personalized strategy based on your genetic profile, you can unlock your potential for lasting weight loss and improved health.

■ *Lean Genes Blueprint* Entry: Reflecting on Genetics 101

Understanding your genetic profile is a critical step in creating a personalized weight loss plan. Take some time to explore that now.

❖ Consider how understanding your genetics could reshape your approach to health.

❖ Which genetic insights are you intrigued to explore more? (Metabolism, fat storage, exercise response?)

❖ Do you have a sense which ones might make a difference for you?

If you are intrigued by genetic weight loss, head to GeneLean360.com to explore genetic testing and begin your journey.

Chapter 7

The Role of Epigenetics in Weight Loss

For so long, I believed my genetics were a life sentence. No matter what I did, every attempt to lose weight seemed to hit an invisible barrier. Then I discovered the science of epigenetics and realized: while we can't change our DNA, we can influence how our genes express themselves. Epigenetics taught me that genes aren't the entire story—our lifestyle choices hold the power to reshape the narrative.

The Science of Epigenetics

Epigenetics is the study of how factors like diet, exercise, stress, and environment influence gene expression without altering the DNA itself.[22] Think of your genetics as a set of instructions and epigenetics as the way you interpret and apply those instructions. Owning a roadmap is one thing; actively choosing the most efficient route to your destination is another.

At the core of epigenetics are chemical tags, often called methyl groups, that attach to DNA and impact which genes are activated or suppressed. Influenced by elements such as the foods we eat, the stress we experience, and even the quality of our sleep, these tags allow us to "switch" certain genes on or off. By consciously adjusting these factors, we can influence our metabolism, appetite regulation, fat storage, and overall energy balance.[23]

Key Epigenetic Influences in Weight Loss

Diet: Nutrient-rich foods, like leafy greens, berries, and omega-3 fatty acids, play a vital role in supporting healthy gene expression.[24] Certain foods can enhance your metabolism or help manage hunger by impacting genes tied to appetite regulation and fat storage. In contrast, highly processed foods and sugary diets can activate gene expressions that encourage fat storage and inflammation.[25]

Exercise: Physical activity goes beyond burning calories. Exercise alters the expression of genes associated with fat metabolism and insulin sensitivity, which is crucial for weight management.[26] Knowing how your body responds to different types of workouts helps you tailor your fitness routine to optimize these genetic benefits.

Stress management: Chronic stress raises cortisol, the stress hormone, which promotes fat storage and disrupts appetite regulation.[27] Stress also affects gene expression, making effective stress management a critical part of an epigenetic-friendly lifestyle.[28] Techniques like deep breathing, meditation, and mindfulness can help balance these effects.

Sleep quality: Quality sleep is foundational for healthy gene expression. Sleep deprivation is linked to genes that increase hunger and cravings, complicating weight management.[29] Restorative sleep supports metabolic health and stress hormone regulation, making it essential for anyone aiming to improve their health.

Epigenetics in Action: From Predisposition to Empowerment

The beauty of epigenetics is its potential to shift us from a place of genetic predisposition to one of empowerment. Someone with a genetic tendency toward fat storage, for example, can, through specific lifestyle choices, switch off or mitigate those genes, enhancing their body's natural weight regulation.

Imagine you've been restricting yourself to extremely low-carbohydrate, low-calorie diets, convinced it's the only path to weight loss. But then, your genetic profile reveals that your body would actually thrive with some pizza or pasta here and there. By embracing these foods in balance, you align your lifestyle with your genetics, allowing you to enjoy your diet while working with—not against—your body's unique needs.

Realign Your Life with Epigenetics

Understanding epigenetics provides a powerful realization: you are not a victim of your genes. Instead, you have the knowledge and tools to harness your genetic potential.

This is just the beginning. In upcoming chapters, we'll dive deep into twelve distinct Genetic Avatars™—from The Fatigue Fighters™ to The Hormone Havoc™—each with unique characteristics, challenges, and actionable steps. These chapters aren't just about providing you with insights; they're designed to help you personalize your approach and turn knowledge into meaningful action.

We'll explore real stories of individuals who have been there before—leveraging their new knowledge about their unique genetic blueprints to transform their bodies and lives. These personalized approaches led to lasting weight loss, improved energy, and a renewed sense of control.

Epigenetics is not about changing who you are; it's about allowing your healthiest self to emerge. As you continue, remember: you have the power to influence your health. You hold the keys to unlocking a path that feels both achievable and transformative.

■ *Lean Genes Blueprint* **Entry: Reflecting on the Role of Epigenetics in Weight Loss**

Even without genetic testing, there are everyday choices you can make to support your health at a genetic level. Reflect on these areas where small, intentional changes can have a lasting impact:

❖ Identify lifestyle habits that could influence your health positively, such as managing stress, prioritizing quality sleep, choosing whole, nutrient-dense foods, or adding movement to your daily routine.

❖ Consider simple, attainable goals that might improve your body's response to these areas. For example, could you add more leafy greens to your diet, set a regular bedtime, or try stress-relief techniques like deep breathing?

By focusing on these changes, you're creating an epigenetic-friendly approach, preparing your body for positive shifts that align with your wellness goals.

DR. PHYLLIS POBEE

PART THREE

THE SECRET TO SUCCESS

DR. PHYLLIS POBEE

Chapter 8

Discovering Your Genetic Avatar

B y now, you've learned that genetics and epigenetics play significant roles in weight management. Your genetic blueprint is a critical piece of the puzzle, one that can unlock new pathways to achieving your health goals. But how can you translate this knowledge into practical steps tailored specifically for *you*? This is where the concept of GeneLean360° Genetic Avatars™ comes into play.

What Are Genetic Avatars™?

Over years of working with clients, I began to see patterns emerge—distinct genetic profiles that reveal how individuals respond differently to diet, exercise, and lifestyle changes. To simplify these complex patterns, I identified twelve Genetic Avatars™, each one representing a unique combination of genetic traits that affect weight loss and overall health.[30]

Genetic Avatars™ are archetypes embodying common genetic variations that influence metabolism, fat storage, appetite, and other factors critical to weight management.[31] By identifying your avatar, you gain insights into your body's specific needs, challenges, and the most effective strategies for you.

Can you have more than one avatar? In short, yes. It's entirely possible that you may identify with more than one of the Genetic Avatars™ in play, as our genetic profiles are rarely discrete.[32] In fact, most clients resonate with one to three Genetic Avatars™, which together form the foundation of their personalized health plan.[33] This is because each individual's genetic profile is unique, and while some genetic markers may be dominant, others can overlap, creating a blend of traits.

Think of your genetics as a layered map, with each layer representing different aspects of how your body functions. One layer might highlight how you respond to carbohydrates, while another shows how you handle stress or process nutrients.[34] When two or three avatars appear, it's often because your genetic profile has variations across these multiple layers, all contributing to your overall health.[35]

From a scientific perspective, each avatar is based on specific genes or SNPs, which are those small variations in DNA we talked about earlier.[36] Since these SNPs can interact, having more than one avatar reflects how your genes collectively affect things like metabolism, appetite, and exercise response.[37]

For example, you might have genes related to both The Fatigue Fighters™ and The Cortisol Carriers™, meaning your body struggles with both energy production and stress, requiring a plan that addresses both. By identifying one to three avatars, we can tailor a protocol that aligns with your unique genetic blend, ensuring a comprehensive approach that addresses multiple factors at once for sustainable results.[38]

The 12 Genetic Avatars™

Here are the 12 Genetic Avatars™:

1. **The Fatigue Fighters™:** You often feel drained and unable to maintain energy, no matter how much you rest, leaving you constantly craving quick fixes just to get through the day.[39]

2. **The Dopamine Drivers™:** Focus and motivation are a daily battle, with impulse control issues that lead to binge eating or difficulty sticking with healthy habits in the long term.[40]

3. **The Cortisol Carriers™:** High stress overwhelms you, triggering intense cravings and weight gain, particularly around your midsection, as your body clings to fat under pressure.[41]

4. **The Inflammatory Overload™:** You struggle with mood swings, fatigue, and energy crashes that seem to come out of nowhere, often worsened by certain foods or environmental factors.[42]

5. **The Sugar Shapers™:** Carbohydrates seem to control your life, leading to spikes, crashes, and constant cravings, leaving you feeling unsteady and dependent on quick sugar fixes.[43]

6. **The Hormone Havoc™:** Hormonal fluctuations make it nearly impossible to find balance, causing intense shifts in mood, energy, and weight, especially during key life changes like menopause.[44]

7. **The Detox Bound™:** Toxins and environmental stressors leave you feeling sluggish and weighed down, making it harder to lose weight and feel energized despite a clean lifestyle.[45]

8. **The Craving Captives™:** Persistent cravings and an inability to feel full have you constantly battling hunger, leading to overeating and frustration with maintaining control over your diet.[46]

9. **The Vascular Vulnerables™:** Cardiovascular issues and low stamina make physical activity challenging, and poor circulation or high blood pressure affect your overall wellness.[47]

10. **The Gut Imbalanced™:** Digestive discomfort, bloating, and nutrient absorption issues leave you feeling heavy and out of sync, impacting both your energy and your weight.[48]

11. **The Carb Converters™:** You're one of the lucky few who can handle carbs well, but balancing intake is still essential to avoid weight gain and maintain steady energy levels.[49]

12. **The Power Performers™:** You thrive on strength and high-intensity workouts, but struggle with recovery and occasional fatigue, especially if your regimen is too demanding.[50]

Why Identifying Your Avatar Matters

Understanding your Genetic Avatars™ empowers you to:
- **Personalize your nutrition plan:** Know which foods fuel your body best and which to minimize.[51]
- **Optimize your exercise routine:** Focus on physical activities that align with your genetic strengths.[52]
- **Manage appetite and cravings:** Learn how your genes affect hunger hormones and adopt strategies to regulate them.[53]
- **Enhance overall well-being:** Address underlying genetic factors that may impact sleep, stress, and energy levels.[54]

The GeneLean360° Difference

No more one-size-fits-all solutions. By embracing your Genetic Avatars™, you're taking control of your health in a way that's aligned with your body's unique blueprint[26]. This personalized approach not only enhances your chances of success, but also makes the journey more enjoyable and sustainable.[55]

With knowledge of your genetic blueprint, you can:

> **Rev up your metabolism:** Targeted nutrients and exercise enhance metabolic pathways influenced by your genes.

> **Reverse weight-loss resistance:** Overcome biological barriers that make weight loss difficult.

> **Achieve effortless weight loss:** Aligning with your body's natural tendencies reduces the struggle and reliance on willpower alone.

The Genetic Weight Loss Journey Begins

You're about to step into one of the most exciting parts of this journey: learning exactly how your unique genetic blueprint can become your greatest asset in reclaiming your body and health.

Get ready to meet real women just like you—women who found their strengths, faced their obstacles, and redefined what success in weight loss means. Each story in the following pages reflects the powerful, individual paths that each of these women took. You'll see that these aren't just "cases" or "profiles"; they're real journeys of rediscovery, growth, and empowerment. As you read, you may find pieces of your own story in theirs.

This part of the book is packed with actionable steps, real-life strategies, and supportive tools designed to make this journey easier. Don't miss the workbook—download it as a companion, and remember that each exercise is crafted to help you personalize what you read here.

For daily inspiration, fresh insights, and more tips, head to my website and join me on Instagram, where we're building a community of women committed to living life fully and confidently.

Let's dive in now. May these stories inspire you and the next steps be uniquely yours.

Lean Genes Blueprint Entry: Discovering Your Genetic Avatar

❖ Consider your past experiences with diet and exercise. Do you notice any patterns that might align with a particular avatar?

❖ Write down what you hope to achieve by personalizing your approach based on your genetic insights.

Chapter 9

The Fatigue Fighters™

For those of us who feel like we're constantly running on empty, meet The Fatigue Fighters™. These are the women who, despite their best efforts, feel drained day after day, their energy lagging behind their goals.

Have you ever wondered why traditional diets leave you exhausted? That was Jessica's experience. Together, we found ways to reignite that inner spark for Jessica, by harnessing small, sustainable changes that made an enormous difference. If your energy dips often, you might just find your own story here. Let's discover what it means to fight fatigue with science, strategy, and self-care.

Phase One: Understanding Jessica's Story

Jessica was a go-getter. She had always been. But lately, at 4'10" and 232 pounds, Jessica felt like she was moving through quicksand. Every morning was a marathon she didn't feel equipped to run. She'd hit the snooze button three, maybe four times, before finally swinging her legs over the side of the bed. The weight of her body seemed to bear down on her bones even as she sat up, and her ankles ached with the first few steps across the room. Her days started with promises to be better—that today she'd eat right, get moving, finally feel energized. But those promises fizzled out as soon as her morning cravings hit.

Jessica had tried it all: cutting carbs, juice cleanses, HIIT, and the latest diet trends that promised quick results. Each new plan started with hope, but quickly led to exhaustion. The low-carb diets left her feeling deprived and mentally foggy. Juice cleanses made her energy plummet, leading to headaches and irritability. High-intensity workouts were the hardest; they drained her so much, she'd collapse on the couch afterward, too tired to do anything else. Despite her best efforts, the scale barely budged, and her clothes grew tighter.

Why these approaches didn't work:

- **Restrictive diets:** Cutting out entire food groups can lead to nutrient deficiencies, especially in essential vitamins and minerals needed for energy production.[56] For someone like Jessica, with genetic variants affecting nutrient absorption, this was particularly counterproductive.

- **Juice cleanses:** While they might offer a temporary reduction in calorie intake, juice cleanses are often high in sugar and lack protein and healthy fats, leading to blood sugar spikes and crashes.[57] This exacerbated Jessica's energy dips and cravings.

- **High-intensity workouts:** Without proper energy and nutrient support, intense exercise can increase stress hormone levels, leading to fatigue and even weight gain around the abdomen.[58]

Mornings were powered by sugar, caffeine, and anything that promised a quick jolt. Lattes, iced coffees with double pumps of caramel, and sugary breakfast bars became her go-to fuel. They'd pick her up for an hour or two, but the crash always came hard and fast. By noon, Jessica was barely holding on, her head nodding at her desk, her mind foggy and distracted. To stay focused, she'd reach for another quick fix—maybe a candy bar from the office stash or another trip to the coffee shop. The vicious cycle felt impossible to escape.

Jessica worked in a high-stakes corporate environment, where the demands never let up. She'd had her eyes on a promotion for years, but lately, she couldn't even gather the courage to apply. Every time she considered it, a voice in her head laughed, "Girl, stop... You'll never make it like this."

Her confidence had been slowly eroding, and she knew part of it was due to the way she felt trapped in her own body. Her suits, once carefully selected to convey power and confidence, now strained at the buttons, and she dreaded the routine of getting dressed. She'd tug at the fabric of her blouse, trying to smooth the lines over her stomach, only to feel the insecurities creep in. Meetings became torture, her focus often drifting to how she was sitting, if her body was spilling out over the chair, if anyone noticed how she shifted uncomfortably to hide her shape.

Her social life had faded, too. She turned down dinners with friends because she knew she'd end up overindulging and regretting it later. Even her family noticed her absence at gatherings, and her mom would call to ask why she didn't bring her "usual bright self" anymore. In truth,

Jessica felt lost, hiding behind excuses and watching from the sidelines as life went on without her. Every day, she felt more like a shell of the ambitious, energetic woman she once was.

One night, as she lay scrolling through TikTok, she came across a video that caught her attention. The creator talked about "getting to the root of your weight issues" and "functional medicine" that looked beyond just calories in, calories out. Jessica was intrigued. She felt seen: the creator talked about chronic fatigue, persistent weight gain, and all these complicated tests.

Jessica saved the video, watched it a few more times, and started researching functional medicine. *Maybe*, she thought, *this is the solution I've been looking for, the approach that will finally explain why every diet I've tried only leaves me drained and discouraged.*

Determined, Jessica scheduled an appointment with a functional medicine doctor. Her first visit was overwhelming. The doctor spoke about hundreds of supplements, chelation therapy, and parasites—things she had never considered before. Jessica left with two pages of supplement recommendations, tests she couldn't pronounce, and the hope that this investment would be the answer.

It wasn't long before the excitement turned into a cumbersome routine. The supplements—twenty in total—were expensive and hard to keep up with. She'd organize them in pill boxes, set alarms, and yet, after months of strict adherence, she still felt just as tired. If anything, she was more overwhelmed, feeling like she'd added one more layer of complexity to her already chaotic life.

Why this approach didn't work:

- **Overwhelming supplement regimen:** Taking numerous supplements without targeted purpose can lead to nutrient imbalances and doesn't address individual genetic needs.[59]

- **Lack of personalization:** Generic functional medicine protocols may not consider specific genetic variants that impact how your body processes nutrients and medications.[60]

- **Compliance challenges:** Complex routines are hard to maintain in the long term, leading to inconsistency and diminished results.[61]

Jessica started to question everything. She'd poured time, energy, and money into this journey and had nothing to show for it but a dwindling bank account and the same drained feeling she'd started with. She saw friends on social media effortlessly losing weight with popular programs, looking vibrant and full of life. In quiet moments, she wondered if she was broken, if there was something deeply different about her that no protocol or supplement could fix.

She wasn't lazy, and she knew she wasn't lacking in motivation. She was just... exhausted. Every step she'd taken felt like sinking deeper into a pit, further from the life and energy she so desperately craved.

Phase Two: Discovering Jessica's Genetic Blueprint

After feeling defeated by her functional medicine approach, Jessica found herself doomscrolling yet again. This time, though, she signed up for a virtual event that gave her goosebumps. It talked about the answer being within her very DNA. She always knew there had to be a reason for why she struggled so much. And so, she took a leap into unlocking her genetic profile with GeneLean360°.

What we uncovered was a revelation—a missing piece of the puzzle that finally explained why so many of her past efforts fell short. Jessica discovered she was part of a genetic group we call **The Fatigue Fighters**™, with a unique set of genetic markers impacting her energy production, nutrient absorption, and metabolism.

Three key genes emerged in Jessica's profile: MTHFR, FUT2, and FTO. Each of these played a crucial role in her body's energy systems:

1. **MTHFR (methylenetetrahydrofolate reductase):** This gene is responsible for a process called methylation, which is essential for converting nutrients like folate and B vitamins into active forms that her body can use.[62] For Jessica, variations in this gene meant her body struggled to utilize these nutrients effectively, leaving her cells starving for energy—even when she was eating nutrient-rich foods or taking supplements.

2. **FUT2 (fucosyltransferase 2):** This gene variation affected her gut health and the way her body absorbed key nutrients, particularly vitamin B12.[63] An inefficient absorption process meant Jessica's body wasn't fully benefiting from the foods and supplements she consumed, explaining the chronic fatigue and the "empty" feeling she often experienced, no matter how much she ate.

3. **FTO (fat mass and obesity-associated protein):**
   Known as the fat gene, this variation can impact
   appetite regulation and fat storage.[64] For Jessica, the
   FTO variant was a double-edged sword—it made
   her crave quick-fix, high-carb foods for an instant
   energy boost, but it also encouraged her body to
   store these extra calories as fat.

Seeing these genetic results was a turning point for
Jessica. The answer to her struggles wasn't a long list of
supplements or the latest trending diet. It was addressing
the root causes of her energy depletion and nutrient
deficiencies. She now understood that her cravings, energy
crashes, and weight struggles weren't a lack of willpower.
They were part of her unique genetic makeup.

Phase Three: Personalized Steps for The Fatigue Fighters™

Armed with a newfound understanding of her genetic
blueprint, Jessica was ready to approach her health and
weight loss journey in a way that aligned with her unique
needs as one of The Fatigue Fighters™. Her transformation
plan was no longer about trying to follow a one-size-fits-all
approach. Instead, it targeted the very core of her energy
depletion and nutrient absorption challenges.

1. GeneLean360° Tailored Nutrition Plan

To optimize her energy and metabolism, Jessica's
nutrition plan focused on foods that would support her
genetic needs and address the nutrient absorption issues
linked to her MTHFR and FUT2 variants.

Macronutrient balance:

- **Moderate protein:** Jessica's meals were structured around moderate protein sources like chicken, fish, tofu, and lentils. These helped with muscle retention and kept her satiated, reducing the need for constant snacking.

- **Complex carbohydrates:** She incorporated low-glycemic carbs like sweet potatoes, quinoa, and oats to stabilize her blood sugar, and to ensure sustained energy, avoiding the spikes and crashes she used to experience. Low-glycemic foods release energy more gradually, helping maintain steady energy and reduce cravings.

- **Healthy fats:** Omega-3-rich fats from sources like salmon, chia seeds, and walnuts supported her brain function, promoted satiety, and provided long-lasting energy.

Why previous diets didn't work:

- **Low-carb diets:** Extreme reduction of carbohydrates can be detrimental for those with FTO variants, leading to increased cravings and decreased energy levels.[65]

- **Juice cleanses:** Lacking in protein and healthy fats, these cleanses can exacerbate blood sugar fluctuations, particularly in individuals sensitive to glycemic variations due to their genetic makeup.[66]

Why this works: This macronutrient balance provided stable energy and avoided the blood sugar crashes to which

Jessica's body, with its FTO variant, was particularly sensitive. With each meal, she was feeding her cells with the type of fuel they needed.

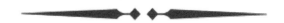

Science Spotlight
Understanding Glycemic Index

The glycemic index, or GI, is a scale that measures how quickly carbohydrates in foods raise blood sugar levels. Foods are rated on a scale from 0 to 100, with higher numbers indicating a faster spike in blood sugar. Low-GI foods (typically 55 or below), like sweet potatoes, quinoa, and oats, release glucose more slowly, leading to gradual, steady energy.

This can be especially beneficial for avatars like The Fatigue Fighters™, who often struggle with energy crashes. By choosing low-GI foods, you can avoid rapid blood sugar spikes and crashes, which helps sustain energy and minimize cravings throughout the day.

Nutrient-dense foods:

o **Leafy greens and cruciferous vegetables:** Spinach, kale, broccoli, and Brussels sprouts became daily staples. These were high in folate, magnesium, and B vitamins, critical nutrients her MTHFR variant struggled to absorb.

o **Berries and citrus fruits:** Packed with antioxidants, these fruits helped in cellular repair and immune function, while their low glycemic index was ideal for Jessica's genetic predisposition.

o **Fortified grains and legumes:** Foods high in B vitamins, such as fortified whole grains and legumes, supported Jessica's energy production and helped address her methylation issues.

Why previous diets didn't work:

> **Restrictive eating plans:** Eliminating whole food groups can deprive the body of essential nutrients, worsening deficiencies caused by genetic variants.[67]

Why this works: By focusing on foods rich in B vitamins and magnesium, Jessica was directly addressing her MTHFR and FUT2 variants, which needed these nutrients in a bioavailable form. This not only improved her energy, but it also reduced her cravings for quick fixes.

Hydration and electrolytes:

o **High water intake:** Jessica began drinking 8-10 glasses of water daily, prioritizing cellular hydration, which reduced her fatigue and kept her energy steady throughout the day.

o **Hydra360° for electrolytes:** To support her hydration and replenish essential electrolytes, Jessica incorporated Hydra360° into her routine. This electrolyte-infused hydration solution provided balanced minerals, helping her stay energized, especially on active days.

Why previous approaches didn't work:

Neglecting hydration: Overlooking the importance of hydration can exacerbate fatigue and hinder metabolic processes.[68]

Why this works: Hydration was crucial for Jessica's cellular energy and nutrient transport. With Hydra360°'s blend of electrolytes, her energy levels improved significantly, directly addressing the fatigue she had experienced due to nutrient imbalances.

2. GeneLean360° Targeted Supplementation™

If you've tried over-the-counter supplements—like the popular B12 in its synthetic form, cyanocobalamin—you may have felt little to no improvement in your energy levels or weight. That's because generic supplements often miss the mark for those with certain genetic variants. These variants can affect how well your body absorbs or utilizes certain nutrients.

Why previous supplements didn't work:

- **Cyanocobalamin inefficiency:** For individuals with the MTHFR gene variant, the body struggles to convert synthetic B12 (cyanocobalamin) into its active form, methylcobalamin, essential for energy production and DNA synthesis.[69]

- **Generic multivitamins:** Often contain forms of nutrients that are not bioavailable to everyone, especially those with absorption issues due to genetic variants.

CoreEnergy360° supplement protocol

Jessica's personalized supplement plan CoreEnergy360° was tailored to work with her unique genetic profile, finally breaking free from the "spray and pray" approach of generic supplements. CoreEnergy360° took a targeted approach, specifically addressing the areas where her body needed support the most.

Key components:

1. Methylated B vitamins and magnesium:
   o Methylated B12 and folate: These bioavailable forms bypass the inefficient conversion process linked to MTHFR SNPs, allowing for direct utilization by the body.[70]
   o Magnesium: Critical in over 300 enzymatic reactions, magnesium supports energy production and reduces fatigue.[71]
2. Probiotics for gut health:
   o Targeted probiotic strains: Specific strains help improve the gut microbiota composition, enhancing nutrient absorption for those with FUT2 variants.[72]

Why this works: By providing nutrients in the forms her body could best utilize, Jessica's metabolism began to work *with* her instead of against her. Her energy became stable, her cravings diminished, and weight loss became less of a daily battle and more of a natural process.

3. GeneLean360° Personalized Fitness Plan

Jessica's fitness routine was structured to build stamina and improve energy without exhausting her limited energy stores.

Why previous workouts didn't work:

- High-intensity overload: Intense workouts can spike cortisol levels and deplete energy reserves, particularly detrimental for those already struggling with fatigue.[73]

- Low- to moderate-intensity cardio:
  - Frequency: 3-4 days per week.
  - Activities: Walking, light jogging, and cycling at a moderate pace.
  - Duration: 30-45 minutes per session.

Why this works: Moderate cardio allowed her to build cardiovascular health without depleting her energy. This approach was essential for her, as a higher intensity might have left her feeling drained and burnt out.

Strength training with a balanced workload:

- **Frequency:** 2-3 days per week.
- **Focus:** Full-body workouts with functional movements like squats, lunges, push-ups, and rows.
- **Reps/sets:** 2-3 sets of 10-12 reps at moderate weights.

Why this works: Building lean muscle mass boosted Jessica's metabolism, helping her body burn more calories efficiently. This balanced approach allowed her to gain strength effectively—without the need for exhausting, high-frequency training—keeping her energized and resilient.

Flexibility and recovery work:

- **Frequency:** 2-3 days per week.
- **Activities:** Gentle yoga, stretching, and foam rolling for 15-20 minutes.

Why this works: Flexibility work supported blood circulation, helped reduce muscle soreness, and promoted a calm recovery, which was particularly helpful given Jessica's nutrient absorption issues and tendency toward fatigue.

Rest and active recovery:

- **Days off:** 1-2 days of rest or light activities like walking.

Why this works: Rest days were critical to allow Jessica's body to recover and rebuild. These helped her avoid burnout, reduced the risk of fatigue, and ultimately supported her consistent progress in weight loss.

Jessica's Transformation and Breakthrough

With her personalized The Fatigue Fighters™ protocol, Jessica's life transformed in ways she had never imagined. The changes came fast. Within weeks, the frantic reach for sugary coffees and mid-morning snacks began to disappear. Her energy began to shift from the kind of jittery bursts she used to get from caffeine and sugar to a steady, calm focus. Gone were the mid-afternoon crashes; instead, she was powering through her days with a clear mind and a newfound sense of stability.

With the cravings gone, Jessica realized her body was responding differently. She no longer needed to strategize to avoid the vending machine or grit her teeth to bypass the sweets in the breakroom. For the first time, she felt fully in control of her hunger, able to make choices that served her without feeling deprived. It was like her body had finally let go of the constant, insatiable hunger that had held her captive for years.

As her energy stabilized, Jessica began to notice changes in her body. Over six months, she lost a remarkable *sixty-three pounds*—a feat she had never come close to achieving before. Her clothes became loose, she moved to smaller sizes, and she felt lighter, both physically and mentally. Her waist, hips, and arms slimmed down as she shed *fourteen inches* across her body, giving her a shape she hadn't seen since her twenties. The weight didn't just melt away; her entire body seemed to reshape, as if she was finally becoming the version of herself that she had always dreamed of.

Jessica noticed she believed in herself more and was regaining her confidence. She even took a bold step forward and decided to apply for that promotion she had long wanted. Walking into that interview, she was no longer held back by insecurities or the sluggishness that had once made her doubt herself. Instead, she radiated confidence and poise. Landing the position felt like proof she had broken free from the fatigue, self-doubt, and constant struggle. She was finally living her life, not just existing day to day.

Outside of work, Jessica was thriving, reconnecting with friends, family, and even her own passions. She said yes to everything she'd been avoiding—dinners with friends, family outings, and even weekend hikes she used to dread. She no longer felt like the tired friend, or the relative who never showed up; she was vibrant, present, and fully engaged in her life. Her transformation became a source of inspiration for those around her.

Through The Fatigue Fighters™ approach, Jessica didn't just lose weight—she gained back her confidence, energy, and joy for life. She was no longer fighting her body; she was thriving in it, empowered and free from the limitations that had once held her back. Her journey was a true breakthrough, not just in her appearance, but in claiming the life she had always deserved.

Jessica's journey shows that persistent fatigue isn't just about willpower—it may be rooted in our genetics. If her story resonates with you, consider exploring your own genetic blueprint to uncover personalized paths to vitality at GeneLean360.com.

▪ Lean *Genes Blueprint* Entry: Uncovering Your Energy Barriers

Turn to your *Lean Genes Blueprint* now to reflect on your own energy struggles and how these may relate to your prior history with dieting.

❖ Have you noticed patterns of fatigue, cravings, or morning energy dips?

❖ Write about the challenges you've faced with traditional diets and why they may have left you feeling drained.

Chapter 10

The Dopamine Drivers™

Kim's story is one of finding freedom from cravings by working with her biology, not against it. For The Dopamine Drivers™, weight loss isn't just about willpower. It's about understanding the genetic tendencies that drive cravings, impulse eating, and reward-seeking. Women like Kim often feel trapped in cycles of intense cravings, but by learning to balance her dopamine needs, Kim transformed her approach.

With a plan tailored to her genetic profile, Kim experienced lasting results, shedding sixty pounds over six months—not through restriction, but by aligning with her body's natural tendencies. This chapter reveals how, like Kim, you can harness your body's unique dopamine pathways to achieve control, balance, and freedom.

Have you ever struggled with compulsive or binge eating? Get ready to meet Kim, a high performer in perimenopause whose weight had gotten out of control. The weight gain, coupled with impulsivity and control issues, made Kim's struggles seem insurmountable. In this chapter, we will break down The Dopamine Drivers™ Genetic Avatar and how understanding her genetic makeup changed her body and her life.

Phase One: Understanding Kim's Story

Kim had crafted her life around control. At forty-two, she was a successful attorney in a top law firm, her career a testament to discipline and perseverance. Her colleagues knew her as the unshakable one—a woman whose sharp mind and dedication had propelled her through countless cases and late nights. Yet, outside the polished walls of her office, Kim was waging a private battle against an enemy she couldn't conquer: her own cravings.

Food had always been her struggle, an area where discipline slipped through her fingers. Each day, she would wake up with renewed determination to control her eating. Black coffee—no sugar, no cream—was her only indulgence as she powered through early morning briefings and client calls. Lunch was an afterthought or sometimes a half-serving of dry salad. By dinner, she would allow herself only a small bowl of soup, convinced that hunger would eventually become bearable.

But by nightfall, after a fourteen-hour day of fighting for others, she'd collapse into her empty apartment. The restraint she'd fought to maintain would understandably crumble, replaced by a ravenous urge that felt beyond her control. Kim would tear through her refrigerator, grabbing everything from stale bread to ice cream, even peanut butter straight from the jar. She ate with an intensity that frightened her, as though trying to fill an emptiness no amount of food could satisfy.

After these binges, she'd sit on the floor, surrounded by empty wrappers, whispering, "What's wrong with me?" She blamed herself for lacking willpower, repeating the same self-recriminations. *Be stronger. Just try harder tomorrow.* But the cycle continued.

Kim's relationships suffered. She excused herself from dinner invitations as she couldn't bear the thought of breaking her restrictive routines or losing control in front of friends. Her once-vibrant social life dwindled, replaced by lonely evenings marked by guilt and shame. She began feeling isolated, even broken, wondering if she'd ever find peace with her body.

Kim had tried it all: strict diets, intense exercise regimens, and over-the-counter supplements that promised to curb cravings. She experimented with low-carb diets, thinking cutting out carbohydrates would help control her appetite. She tried HIIT classes, hoping to burn off the excess weight. She even took popular appetite suppressants she found online. Yet, none of these approaches provided lasting relief; in fact, they often made her cravings worse.

Why these approaches didn't work:

- **Restrictive diets:** Eliminating entire food groups, such as carbohydrates, can actually lower serotonin and dopamine levels in the brain, increasing cravings and mood swings.[74] For someone like Kim with genetic variations affecting dopamine regulation, this exacerbates the problem.

- **Intense exercise regimens:** While exercise can boost dopamine temporarily, excessive high-intensity workouts can lead to increased cortisol, which may promote weight gain and increase cravings.[75]

- **Over-the-counter appetite suppressants:** Generic supplements often don't account for individual genetic differences. Without targeting the specific dopamine pathways affected by Kim's genetic makeup, these products offered little benefit.[76]

One day, Kim shared with me how she ran into Rina, an old friend from college and a former client of mine. Rina looked radiant, healthy in a way that startled Kim. The last she'd heard, Rina had also been struggling with weight. Yet here she was, seemingly transformed. When Kim asked how, Rina shared something that took her by surprise.

"Genetic testing with GeneLean360°. I realized it wasn't just about willpower. I learned my body has specific genetic factors affecting my eating habits and cravings. Now, instead of fighting myself, I know what works for me."

Intrigued, Kim pressed for details, and Rina recommended she try GeneLean360°. For the first time, a glimmer of hope surfaced. What if her struggles weren't solely about discipline? What if there was a reason she'd been fighting so hard with no lasting results?

That night, instead of her usual binge, Kim researched GeneLean360° and watched a Reel that shared how genetic markers could reveal underlying challenges with dopamine regulation, appetite, and even emotional control. As she read, tears began to fall—she felt like her hidden struggles were being laid bare.

Kim booked a consultation, daring to believe that maybe, just maybe, her life could change.

Phase Two: Discovering Kim's Genetic Blueprint

On the day we reviewed Kim's genetic results, I could see the apprehension and hope in her eyes. She leaned forward, searching my face as I opened her report.

"Kim," I began gently, "your results show that you fall into a group we call The Dopamine Drivers™."

Her eyes widened with curiosity and a hint of relief. "What does that mean?"

"It means that certain genetic markers—specifically in the DRD2, COMT, and SLC6A3 genes—impact how your body regulates dopamine," I explained.[77] "Dopamine is a neurotransmitter crucial for motivation, impulse control, and feeling rewarded. But variations in these genes can lower dopamine production or receptor sensitivity, making it difficult for your brain to feel 'rewarded' through everyday activities. Your brain, in turn, seeks external rewards, like food, to compensate."

Kim's shoulders slumped in relief. "So, it's not just that I lack willpower?"

"Not at all," I reassured her. "Your behaviors are biologically driven. It's not about discipline, but about working with your genetic tendencies. The good news is that we can create a tailored plan to help stabilize your dopamine levels and give you the tools you need."

As we went through her genetic results, I explained how each gene played a role:

- **DRD2:** This gene influences dopamine receptor density. Lower receptor density often results in lower dopamine activity, making it harder for her brain to feel rewarded. This gene variant meant Kim was more likely to seek dopamine through external rewards like food.[78]

- **COMT:** This gene breaks down dopamine. Kim's variant made her break it down faster than average, leading to brief dopamine spikes followed by sharp drops. This explained her pattern of intense cravings and quick mood dips.[79]

- **SLC6A3:** This gene regulates dopamine transport. Variations here can lead to lower dopamine levels in certain parts of the brain, reducing impulse control and intensifying her need for reward-seeking behavior.[80]

Why previous approaches didn't work based on these SNPs:

- **Restrictive diets:** For someone with a COMT variant leading to rapid dopamine breakdown, cutting out carbohydrates can further reduce dopamine availability, intensifying cravings and mood swings.[81]

- **Intense exercise regimens:** Excessive exercise can temporarily boost dopamine, but may also increase dopamine breakdown in those with COMT variants, leading to greater deficits later.[82]

- **Over-the-counter supplements:** Generic appetite suppressants or dopamine boosters don't account for variations in DRD2 and SLC6A3, making them ineffective for improving dopamine receptor sensitivity or transport in individuals like Kim.[83]

Hearing these explanations brought a newfound lightness to Kim's face. For years, she had blamed herself, not realizing that her struggles had a biological basis.

"So, what do we do?" she asked, eager yet cautious.

"Now that we understand what's happening, we can create a plan that aligns with your body's needs," I told her. "With the right nutrition, supplementation, and fitness plan, we'll help your brain feel rewarded and balanced, so you don't have to rely on food binges." For the first time, Kim felt empowered. She wasn't fighting against herself—she was finally working with her body.

Phase Three: Personalized Steps for The Dopamine Drivers™

With a clear understanding of her unique dopamine-driven challenges, Kim embarked on a plan tailored to her genetic profile.

1. GeneLean360° Tailored Nutrition Plan

To support her dopamine regulation and prevent binge eating, Kim's nutrition plan was designed to keep her energy stable and minimize dopamine "crashes."

Protein-rich foods to support dopamine production:

o **Lean proteins:** Kim's meals now included chicken, turkey, eggs, lean beef, tofu, and tempeh to provide tyrosine, an amino acid that supports dopamine production.[84]

o **Protein at every meal:** She ensured protein was a staple in each meal, especially breakfast, to set a stable foundation for the day.

Why: Protein-rich foods are essential for dopamine synthesis, helping Kim improve focus and motivation while reducing impulsive eating.

Complex carbohydrates for mood stability:

- ○ **Low-glycemic carbs:** Kim chose oats, quinoa, sweet potatoes, and whole grains to maintain steady energy levels.

- ○ **Avoiding simple sugars:** Refined sugars and high-glycemic carbs were limited to prevent spikes and crashes that could exacerbate her cravings.[85]

Why: Stable blood sugar levels were essential for Kim, as it helped stabilize her mood and reduced her need for dopamine-boosting foods.

Healthy fats to support brain health:

- ○ **Omega-3-rich foods:** Including fatty fish, chia seeds, and walnuts for brain health and inflammation reduction.[86]

- ○ **Moderate healthy fats:** Avocado, almonds, and olive oil promoted satiety without triggering cravings.

Why: Omega-3s improved dopamine receptor sensitivity, helping Kim feel more focused and balanced.

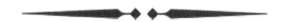

Science Spotlight

Understanding Dopamine and Diet

Dopamine is synthesized from tyrosine, an amino acid found in protein-rich foods. Consuming adequate protein ensures a steady supply of tyrosine for dopamine production.[87] Additionally, complex carbohydrates facilitate the entry of tyrosine into the brain by stimulating insulin release, which helps in the amino acid transport process.[88] Balancing protein with complex carbs is essential for The Dopamine Drivers™ to maintain optimal dopamine levels and control cravings.

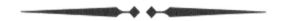

Nutrient-dense, dopamine-supportive foods:

- o **Green tea:** Contains L-theanine, which can enhance dopamine production.[89]

- o **Bananas:** Rich in vitamin B6 and tyrosine, supporting dopamine synthesis.

- o **Dark chocolate:** Contains phenylethylamine, promoting dopamine release (in moderation).

Why: These foods naturally boost dopamine levels, helping Kim feel more satisfied and less reliant on overeating for pleasure.

Hydration:

- o **Adequate water intake:** Kim aimed for at least eight glasses of water daily to support overall metabolic function and neurotransmitter synthesis.

Why: Proper hydration is essential for optimal brain function and can help reduce false hunger cues.[90]

2. GeneLean360° Targeted Supplementation™

If you've tried over-the-counter supplements—like generic dopamine boosters or appetite suppressants—and still find yourself battling cravings and weight gain, it's not your fault.

Why over-the-counter supplements often fail:

- **Generic formulations:** Most off-the-shelf supplements aren't designed to address specific genetic variations. They may contain forms of nutrients that aren't effectively utilized by your body due to SNPs in genes like COMT, DRD2, **and** SLC6A3.[91]

- **Ineffective dosages:** Without personalized dosing, you might not get the therapeutic levels needed to make a real difference.

- **Overlooked nutrient interactions:** Some supplements may not consider how different nutrients interact, potentially counteracting each other's effects.

FocusBalance360° supplement protocol

Kim's personalized supplementation plan was tailored to her genetic profile and included FocusBalance360°, directly addressing her dopamine regulation issues.

Key components:

L-Tyrosine and Mucuna Pruriens Extract

o **Why this works:** These ingredients act as precursors to dopamine, enhancing its production and availability. Together, they support focus, motivation, and reward pathways, which are crucial for managing cravings and impulsive behaviors.

This unique blend stabilizes dopamine and serotonin levels, promoting feelings of reward and satisfaction without relying on high-calorie foods, helping individuals like Kim stay on track with her health and weight loss goals.[92,93]

o **Why generic supplements don't work:** For individuals with dopamine-related SNPs in DRD2 or SLC6A3, low dopamine sensitivity makes it hard to feel rewarded by everyday experiences. This can lead to seeking external sources of comfort, such as food. Our blend of L-Tyrosine and Mucuna Pruriens directly targets dopamine production and receptor sensitivity, effectively addressing genetic dopamine deficiencies and promoting a balanced reward response.[94,95]

2. 5-HTP and Gamma-Aminobutyric Acid (GABA)

o **Why this works:** 5-HTP is a precursor to serotonin, which regulates mood, appetite, and impulse control. Combined with GABA, which promotes relaxation and reduces overstimulation, these ingredients work together to stabilize mood and reduce emotional triggers for cravings. This combination supports a calm, focused mental state, helping prevent overeating and impulsive behaviors.[96,97]

o **Why generic supplements didn't work**: Generic supplements often lack the synergy between serotonin and GABA support, leading to inadequate mood stabilization. For individuals with stress-induced cravings or serotonin-related SNPs, this deficiency leaves emotional triggers unresolved, making it harder to stay on track.[98,99]

3. DiMagnesium Malate, Zinc, and L-Theanine

o **Why this works**: DiMagnesium Malate provides bioavailable magnesium to support enzymatic reactions involved in neurotransmitter synthesis and calm the nervous system.[100] Zinc supports dopamine production and receptor function, while L-Theanine promotes relaxation without drowsiness, balancing stress and focus[101,102]. Together, these nutrients enhance neurotransmitter efficiency, reduce stress-induced cravings, and improve focus and mental clarity.

o **Why generic supplements didn't work**: Generic supplements often use less bioavailable forms of magnesium and zinc, leading to poor absorption and insufficient support for neurotransmitter activity. Additionally, they lack L-Theanine's ability to modulate stress and focus, making them less effective at addressing stress-related eating behaviors.[103, 104, 105]

Why this targeted approach works:

- **Addresses genetic variations directly:** By tailoring supplementation to her specific SNPs, Kim's protocol enhanced dopamine production, receptor sensitivity, and slowed down dopamine breakdown.

- **Bypasses metabolic roadblocks:** Using bioactive nutrient forms ensured her body could utilize them effectively, overcoming absorption issues common with generic supplements.

- **Reduces cravings and improves mood:** Stabilizing dopamine levels helped Kim feel more satisfied and less prone to impulsive eating.

3. GeneLean360° Personalized Fitness Plan

Kim's fitness routine was designed to provide natural dopamine boosts without overwhelming her system.

Why previous workouts didn't work:

- **High-intensity overload:** Intense workouts can temporarily spike dopamine, but may lead to crashes, especially for those with rapid dopamine degradation due to COMT variants.[106]

Balanced exercise routine:

- **Moderate-intensity cardio:**

  o **Frequency:** 3-4 days per week.

  o **Activities:** Brisk walking, cycling, dance classes.

  o **Duration:** 30-45 minutes per session.

Why: Moderate cardio stimulates dopamine release without causing excessive stress on the body, helping improve mood and motivation.[107]

- **Strength training:**

  o **Frequency:** 2-3 days per week.

  o **Focus:** Full-body workouts using compound movements like squats, lunges, and rows.

Why: Resistance training enhances neurotransmitter function and promotes endorphin release, contributing to overall well-being.[108]

- **Mind-body practices:**

  o **Frequency:** 2-3 days per week.

  o **Activities:** Yoga, Pilates, tai chi.

Why: These practices reduce stress hormones and improve dopamine receptor sensitivity, aiding in impulse control and emotional balance.[109]

4. Mindfulness and Stress Management

Why this is essential:

- **Stress increases dopamine depletion:** Chronic stress can exacerbate dopamine imbalance, intensifying cravings and impulsivity.[110]

Strategies implemented:

- **Meditation and deep breathing:**

  o **Benefit:** Reduces cortisol levels and supports neurotransmitter balance.

- **Journaling:**

  o **Benefit:** Helps identify emotional triggers for cravings, allowing for proactive management.

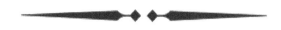

Science Spotlight

Understanding Dopamine Dysregulation and its Impact on Cravings and Impulsivity

For individuals with attention deficit hyperactivity disorder (ADHD), dopamine dysregulation is often at the core of many challenges, including impulsivity, cravings, and emotional eating.

ADHD is commonly associated with variations in dopamine-related genes, such as COMT, DRD2, and SLC6A3, which affect dopamine levels, receptor sensitivity, and dopamine breakdown in the brain. This imbalance can make it difficult for the brain to feel fully rewarded or satisfied, leading to behaviors aimed at boosting dopamine levels, like reaching for high-reward foods.

This dopamine imbalance can have several key effects:

- **Increased cravings:** Since dopamine is crucial for feeling rewarded, individuals with ADHD may experience intense cravings for sugary, carb-rich, or high-fat foods, which provide a quick dopamine boost. These cravings are the brain's attempt to self-regulate dopamine and create a sense of satisfaction or pleasure.

- **Impulsivity in eating:** The impulsive tendencies associated with ADHD can make it challenging to resist food temptations. The drive to seek immediate rewards often overpowers logical thinking about long-term goals, making healthy eating and portion control difficult.

- **Emotional eating as self-regulation:** Many people with ADHD turn to food for comfort and emotional regulation, as it can temporarily improve mood and focus by boosting dopamine. This coping mechanism can lead to overeating and weight gain, as the brain continuously seeks these quick fixes.

Understanding these dopamine-driven tendencies is essential for developing a sustainable approach to weight loss and wellness.

By focusing on targeted supplementation, nutrition, and balanced lifestyle choices that support dopamine stability, those with ADHD can better manage cravings, improve impulse control, and create a healthy relationship with food that works *with* their biology.

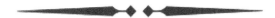

Kim's Transformation and Breakthrough

In the early weeks, adjusting was tough, but with each day, Kim felt stronger. Her cravings subsided, replaced by a sense of satisfaction from nutrient-rich meals. Her energy stabilized, and the pull toward binge eating faded.

Over six months, Kim lost *sixty pounds*—not through restrictive dieting but through balance. Her relationships revived as she accepted invitations, sharing meals without fear. Her career soared with her mind sharper and more focused. Kim had finally found control, not by fighting herself, but by understanding and nurturing her body.

Kim's journey shows the power of understanding your genetic blueprint. For those facing similar challenges with impulsivity and emotional eating, remember: the answers lie within. Visit GeneLean360.com to unlock your genetic potential and achieve freedom from cravings.

▪ *Lean Genes Blueprint* Entry: Mapping Out Your Cravings and Focus Patterns

Reflect on your relationship with cravings, focus, and impulsivity.

- ❖ Have there been times when you felt out of control or wondered if willpower alone was enough?

- ❖ Write down any recurring triggers for binge eating or motivation lapses, and consider how a plan tailored to your unique dopamine needs might look.

Chapter 11

The Cortisol Carriers™

M aya's story shows that understanding your stress response can be the key to reclaiming your body. For The Cortisol Carriers™, stress often drives weight gain and exhaustion, and traditional approaches may only provide temporary relief. Maya's journey began when she discovered how her cortisol spikes were rooted in her genetics, not just her lifestyle. Armed with this insight, she embraced a tailored plan and, over six months, shed twenty pounds, particularly around her midsection. This chapter reveals how, like Maya, you can work with your body to manage stress, support your health, and achieve lasting transformation.

Have you ever felt that stress is sabotaging your weight-loss efforts? Meet Maya, a high-achieving professional and mother who found herself trapped in a cycle of stress and weight gain. Despite her best efforts, traditional approaches only offered temporary relief. In this chapter, we'll explore how understanding her genetic makeup as one of The Cortisol Carriers™ allowed Maya to break free from stress-induced weight gain and transform her life.

Phase One: Understanding Maya's Story

Maya stared at her computer, the cursor blinking on her screen as emails poured in. It was only Monday morning, but already the week loomed over her like a mountain she wasn't sure she could climb. At forty-three Maya was a successful interior designer in New York City, managing a growing business, two teenage boys, and a whirlwind of client demands. Yet, beneath her polished exterior, she was unraveling.

Each day was a marathon. She'd wake before dawn, her mind racing with the to-do list she could never quite catch up with. Her mornings started with coffee—a ritual she relied on to clear the fog of exhaustion. But it wasn't enough. Despite her efforts to control her diet and exercise regularly, Maya found herself constantly on edge, reaching for quick fixes to power through the day: another cup of coffee, a sugary snack from the office kitchen, or something salty to soothe her nerves. The scale wasn't her friend, either—no matter what she tried, her weight crept up, particularly around her midsection.

Maya had explored everything in her search for relief from the stress and fatigue. She started with meditation apps, but her mind wandered within minutes, refusing to quiet. Then, after a particularly challenging week, she booked an acupuncture session, hoping the ancient practice might unlock some hidden well of calm within her. As she lay on the treatment table, needles carefully placed along her body, she allowed herself a rare moment of stillness. But as she left the clinic, her phone buzzed with emails, and the feeling of calm was replaced by a familiar wave of anxiety.

Next, she tried herbal remedies she'd read about online—passionflower, valerian root, and lavender teas stocked her pantry. But none seemed to touch the root of her stress. Even an extensive retreat in upstate New York, which involved yoga and mindfulness exercises, only left her feeling temporarily calm. Once she returned to the city, her stress spiked all over again.

Why these approaches didn't work:

- **Lack of personalization:** Generic stress-relief methods don't account for individual genetic differences in stress response.[111]

- **Temporary solutions:** Practices like meditation and acupuncture can provide short-term relief but may not address underlying genetic predispositions to heightened stress.[112]

- **Ineffective for genetic variations:** Herbal remedies and mindfulness techniques may not sufficiently impact cortisol regulation in individuals with specific genetic variations affecting stress hormones.[113]

After a series of sleepless nights, Maya felt desperation creeping in. She searched "belly fat" and saw a Reel where I was discussing stress-induced weight gain and mentioned the role of cortisol in the body. She told me she watched it ten times, because it felt like it was her story on the screen.

Intrigued, Maya visited the website, where she learned about GeneLean360° and how personalized weight loss could be based on genetic testing. She scheduled a consultation, cautiously hopeful that there might be a scientific explanation for her struggles—and, better yet, a solution.

Phase Two: Discovering Maya's Genetic Blueprint

During our genetic test session, I could see the mix of skepticism and hope in Maya's eyes. She shared her struggles, and I listened attentively before reviewing her genetic test results.

"Maya, your results indicate that you fall into a group we call The Cortisol Carriers™."

She looked at me curiously. "What does that mean?"

"It means that certain genetic markers—specifically in the MAOA, GABRA2, HTR1A, and NR3C1 genes—affect how your body responds to stress," I explained.[114,115,116,117] "These genes influence your cortisol levels, neurotransmitter balance, and stress resilience. Variations in these genes can lead to higher cortisol spikes when you're under stress, which can cause weight gain, especially around the abdomen, and increase cravings for comfort foods."

Maya sighed deeply. "That explains so much. I always thought it was just my hectic life."

"While lifestyle plays a role, your genetics predispose you to a heightened stress response," I continued. "The good news is, now that we understand this, we can create a personalized plan to help manage your cortisol levels and reduce the impact of stress on your weight and overall health."

As we delved deeper into her results, I highlighted how each gene contributed to her experience:

- **MAOA (monoamine oxidase A):** This gene affects the breakdown of neurotransmitters like serotonin and dopamine. Variations can lead to increased anxiety and stress sensitivity.

- **GABRA2 (gamma-aminobutyric acid type A receptor alpha2 subunit):** This gene influences GABA receptors, critical for calming the nervous system. Certain variants can reduce GABA activity, leading to heightened stress responses.

- **HTR1A (5-hydroxytryptamine receptor 1A):** This gene impacts serotonin signaling. Variations can affect mood regulation and stress resilience.

- **NR3C1 (glucocorticoid receptor gene):** This gene affects cortisol receptor sensitivity. Certain variants can make the body less efficient at regulating cortisol levels, leading to prolonged stress responses.

Why previous approaches didn't work based on these SNPs:

- **Generic stress-relief methods:** For someone with variations in **MAOA** and **GABRA2**, generic meditation and relaxation techniques may not sufficiently impact neurotransmitter imbalances, making it hard to achieve lasting calm.[118]

- **Herbal remedies:** Without targeting specific genetic pathways, standard herbal supplements may not effectively regulate cortisol levels influenced by **NR3C1** variations.[119]

- **Mindfulness practices:** While beneficial, these practices alone may not address the heightened stress sensitivity due to **HTR1A** variations.[120]

Understanding these genetic factors was a revelation for Maya. "So, my body is essentially wired to react more intensely to stress?"

"Exactly," I affirmed. "But with targeted nutrition, supplementation, and lifestyle strategies, we can help balance your stress response."

Maya's face lit up with a newfound determination. "I'm ready to make changes."

Phase Three: Personalized Steps for The Cortisol Carriers™

Armed with her new understanding, Maya was ready to approach her health and weight loss journey in a way that aligned with her unique needs as one of The Cortisol Carriers™. Her transformation plan was no longer about generic stress management. It was about targeting the root causes of her heightened stress response.

1. GeneLean360° Tailored Nutrition Plan

To support adrenal health and stabilize blood sugar, Maya's nutrition plan focused on calming, nutrient-dense foods.

What Maya tried before and why it didn't work:

High caffeine intake: Maya relied on multiple cups of coffee to combat fatigue.

Why it didn't work: Caffeine can increase cortisol production, exacerbating stress and leading to energy crashes.[121]

Sugary and salty snacks: She reached for quick fixes to soothe her nerves.

Why it didn't work: High-glycemic and processed foods cause blood sugar spikes and crashes, triggering cortisol release and increasing abdominal fat storage.[122]

Skipping meals: Her busy schedule led her to skip meals or eat irregularly.

Why it didn't work: Irregular eating can disrupt blood sugar balance, leading to cortisol spikes and increased stress.[123]

What did work:

- **Balanced macros with focus on protein and healthy fats:**

  o **Moderate protein: Lean proteins:** Incorporating chicken, turkey, tofu, eggs, and fatty fish, like salmon.

Why: Protein helps stabilize energy levels and supports muscle retention, preventing muscle loss due to high cortisol.[124]

  o **Healthy fats: Omega-3 fatty acids**, including salmon, chia seeds, and flaxseeds. And **Monounsaturated fats**, like avocado and olive oil.

Why: Healthy fats support brain health and improve stress resilience by reducing inflammation.[125]

○ **Low to moderate carbohydrates,** including complex carbs: Sweet potatoes, brown rice, and quinoa.

Why: These provide steady energy without spiking blood sugar, preventing cortisol spikes associated with high-glycemic foods.[126]

- **Adrenal-supportive foods:**

○ **Leafy greens and cruciferous vegetables,** including spinach, kale, broccoli, Brussels sprouts.

Why: Rich in magnesium and B vitamins, essential for combating stress effects and supporting adrenal function.[127]

○ **Vitamin C-rich foods,** including bell peppers, oranges, strawberries, kiwis.

Why: Vitamin C supports adrenal health and reduces oxidative stress, helping lower cortisol levels.[128]

○ **Magnesium-rich foods,** like pumpkin seeds, almonds, dark chocolate.

Why: Magnesium promotes muscle relaxation and a sense of calm, counteracting stress.[129]

- **Anti-inflammatory and cortisol-reducing herbs and spices:**

○ **Incorporate adaptogens** like turmeric, ginger, cinnamon, ashwagandha, holy basil.

Why: Adaptogens help the body adapt to stress and balance cortisol levels.[130]

○ **Green tea and herbal teas,** like matcha, chamomile, holy basil tea.

Why: These teas contain L-theanine and other compounds that promote relaxation and reduce cortisol.[131]

▪ **Controlled meal timing with evening focus:**

○ **Balanced breakfasts,** which include protein, complex carbs, and healthy fats.

Why: Starting the day with a balanced meal helps stabilize blood sugar and sets a calm tone for the day.[132]

○ **Lighter evening meal,** with a focus on protein and vegetables and limited carbohydrates.

Why: A lighter dinner can prevent nighttime cortisol spikes and improve sleep quality[ibid].

Why this works when everything else did not:

By focusing on foods that stabilize blood sugar and support adrenal function, Maya's nutrition plan directly addressed her genetic predisposition to heightened cortisol responses. This approach helped reduce stress-induced cravings, particularly for sugary and salty snacks, and promoted a sense of calm energy throughout the day.

2. GeneLean360° Targeted Supplementation™

If you've tried over-the-counter supplements like generic stress-relief formulas or herbal teas without significant improvement, it's not your fault.

Why over-the-counter supplements often fail:

- **Generic formulations:** Most off-the-shelf stress supplements don't account for individual genetic variations affecting stress hormones like cortisol.

- **Ineffective dosages:** Without personalized dosing, you might not receive therapeutic levels needed to impact cortisol regulation.

- **Overlooked nutrient interactions:** Some supplements may not consider how different ingredients interact, potentially counteracting each other's effects.

Rebalance360° supplement protocol

Maya's personalized supplementation plan was tailored to her genetic profile and included Rebalance360°, directly addressing her cortisol regulation issues.

Key components:

1. **Ashwagandha root extract:**

   o **Benefit:** An adaptogen known to reduce cortisol levels and anxiety, enhancing stress resilience.[133]

   o **Why generic supplements didn't work:** Over-the-counter adaptogens may not be standardized for potency or combined with other supportive nutrients.

2. **Phosphatidylserine:**

   o **Benefit:** It helps reduce cortisol levels and improve cognitive function under stress.[134]

o **Why this works:** Phosphatidylserine supports the body's ability to manage cortisol spikes, which is essential for individuals with NR3C1 variations affecting cortisol receptor sensitivity.

3. **L-theanine:**

o **Benefit:** It promotes relaxation without drowsiness by increasing GABA and serotonin levels.[135]

o **Why generic supplements didn't work:** Standard formulations may not provide sufficient L-theanine to impact GABA activity, crucial for those with GABRA2 variations.

4. **Rhodiola rosea root extract:**

o **Benefit:** Rhodiola rosea root extract improves energy, reduces fatigue, and helps the body adapt to stress.[136]

o **Why this works:** Rhodiola supports neurotransmitter balance, aiding those with MAOA and HTR1A variations in regulating mood and stress response.

Why this targeted approach worked when everything else did not:

- **Addresses genetic variations directly:** By tailoring supplementation to her specific SNPs, Maya's protocol enhanced cortisol regulation and neurotransmitter balance.

- **Bypasses metabolic roadblocks:** Using standardized, bioactive forms ensured her body could utilize the supplements effectively.

- **Reduces stress and improves mood:** Stabilizing cortisol levels helped Maya feel calmer and less prone to stress-induced cravings.

3. GeneLean360° Personalized Fitness Plan

Maya's fitness routine focused on reducing cortisol levels and incorporating stress-relieving activities.

What Maya tried before and why it didn't work:

- **High-intensity workouts:** Maya engaged in intense exercise sessions, believing they would help her lose weight.

  Why it didn't work: High-intensity workouts can increase cortisol levels, exacerbating stress and leading to weight gain, especially in those with **NR3C1** variations.[137]

- **Irregular exercise routine:** Due to her busy schedule, her workouts were sporadic.

  Why it didn't work: Inconsistent exercise doesn't provide the regular stress relief needed to manage cortisol levels effectively.

What did work:

- **Low to moderate-intensity cardio:**
  - **Frequency:** 3-4 times per week.

- o **Activities:** Walking in nature, gentle cycling, swimming.
- o **Duration:** 30-45 minutes per session.

Why: Moderate cardio releases endorphins that counteract cortisol without putting excessive strain on the body.[138]

- **Gentle strength training:**
  - o **Frequency:** 2-3 times per week.
  - o **Exercises:** Lunges, squats, rows, push-ups with controlled movements.
  - o **Reps/sets:** 2-3 sets of 8-12 reps using moderate weights.

Why: Builds lean muscle mass to boost metabolism without overloading the adrenal system.[139]

- **Mind-body exercises for stress reduction:**
  - o **Frequency:** 2-3 times per week.
  - o **Activities:** Yoga, tai chi, Pilates.
  - o **Duration:** 20-30 minutes per session.

Why these were selected:

- **Enhanced GABA activity:** Practices like yoga and tai chi have been shown to increase GABA levels, directly benefiting those with GABRA2 variations.[140]

- **Accessibility and effectiveness:** Unlike meditation apps that Maya struggled with, these physical practices combine movement with mindfulness, making it easier for her to stay engaged and achieve relaxation.

- **Reduced cortisol levels:** These exercises are effective in lowering cortisol and improving stress resilience, aligning with Maya's genetic needs.[141]

- **Rest days with active recovery:**

  o **Frequency:** 1-2 rest days per week.

  o **Activities:** Light stretching, leisurely walks, foam rolling.

  Why: Active recovery promotes muscle relaxation and circulation without raising cortisol levels, essential for recovery and stress management.[142]

Why this works: By shifting to a fitness routine that emphasizes stress reduction and cortisol management, Maya was able to exercise without triggering cortisol spikes. The incorporation of mind-body practices provided dual benefits for her physical and mental health, directly addressing her genetic predispositions.

Maya's Transformation and Breakthrough

As Maya embraced her personalized plan, she began to notice significant changes. Within weeks, her energy levels improved, and the brain fog that once plagued her started to lift. By focusing on balanced meals and incorporating adrenal-supportive foods, she no longer relied on multiple cups of coffee to get through the day.

Her sleep quality improved as she practiced mindfulness exercises and adhered to a lighter evening meal. She woke up feeling more refreshed, which positively impacted her mood and productivity at work.

The incorporation of Rebalance360° supplements further enhanced her stress resilience. She felt calmer in high-pressure situations and noticed that her usual stress-induced cravings diminished. The weight that had stubbornly clung to her midsection began to decrease, and over six months, she lost *twenty pounds*.

Maya's family life improved as well. She was more present with her children and had the energy to engage in activities with them. Her husband noticed the positive changes and supported her journey wholeheartedly.

At work, colleagues commented on her radiant appearance and calm demeanor. She tackled projects with renewed focus and creativity, no longer feeling overwhelmed by stress.

Maya realized that understanding and working with her genetic blueprint was the key to unlocking a healthier, happier life. She was no longer fighting against her body's natural tendencies, but nurturing them in a way that promoted balance and well-being.

Maya's journey demonstrates the profound impact that understanding your genetic makeup can have on your health and quality of life. If you find yourself struggling with stress, unexplained weight gain, and fatigue, consider exploring your own genetic blueprint. By tailoring your nutrition, supplementation, and fitness strategies to your unique needs as one of The Cortisol Carriers™, you can manage stress more effectively and achieve lasting transformation.

If Maya's story resonates with you, consider exploring your own genetic makeup to uncover personalized strategies for managing stress and achieving your health goals. Visit GeneLean360.com to begin your journey toward balance and empowerment.

◼ *Lean Genes Blueprint* Entry: Identifying Your Stress Triggers

Think about how stress has impacted your weight and health journey.

❖ Are there specific stressors or patterns in your life that lead to emotional eating or exhaustion?

❖ Reflect on past attempts to manage stress and where a tailored approach could better address your cortisol responses.

Head to geneticweightlossbook.com/resources to access your workbook and explore personalized strategies for stress management.

Chapter 12

The Inflammatory Overload™

Chioma's story reminds us that even the most determined efforts can feel frustrating without a personalized approach. For those like Chioma with The Inflammatory Overload™ profile, chronic inflammation makes weight loss an uphill battle, often leaving them fatigued and discouraged. Once Chioma began working with her body's needs, her progress felt like a breakthrough. By embracing a plan tailored to reduce inflammation, Chioma lost *eighteen pounds* in four months—and even came off her blood-pressure medication. This chapter will show you how targeted changes can make lasting wellness feel achievable.

Have you ever felt, no matter how hard you try, your body resists weight loss? Meet Chioma, a vibrant woman who found herself trapped in a cycle of fatigue and weight gain despite her best efforts. In this chapter, we'll explore how understanding her genetic makeup as The Inflammatory Overload™ allowed Chioma to overcome her challenges and transform her health.

Phase One: Understanding Chioma's Story

Chioma had always been deeply connected to her cultural roots through food and community. Born to Nigerian parents and raised in Texas, she embraced her heritage through flavorful dishes like jollof rice, egusi soup, and smoked fish, balanced with a love for Southern soul food like fried chicken and cornbread. Lately, though, this joyful relationship with food had become clouded by discomfort and frustration. Despite her best efforts, every meal seemed to leave her feeling more bloated, fatigued, and unsettled.

At thirty-five, Chioma decided it was time to make a serious commitment to her health. She registered at the premium gym in her neighborhood, and invested five figures in a six-month membership, including personal training. Five days a week, she would push herself through intense circuits, weightlifting, and high-energy cardio sessions. Yet, at the end of six months, Chioma was devastated to find she had actually gained five pounds.

Feeling defeated, Chioma began to question everything. She'd been putting in hours of sweat equity, practically living on kale salads, and restricting herself in every way possible. Yet no matter what she did, her body seemed to resist. Friends and family had even started to comment on her lingering fatigue and visible swelling around her face and joints.

It was around this time that Chioma read an article in *Women's World* about me and my GeneLean360° program, which focused on genetic testing to uncover hidden weight loss barriers. For the first time, Chioma felt a glimmer of hope. Perhaps her struggles weren't a matter of willpower or motivation, but rather a genetic factor she hadn't considered. Intrigued and ready to try something new, she booked a consultation with me.

Part Two: Discovering Chioma's Genetic Blueprint

When Chioma and I met to discuss her genetic results, she arrived with equal parts excitement and apprehension. She was ready for answers but unsure of what to expect.

"Chioma, your results suggest that you fall into a genetic profile we call The Inflammatory Overload™," I shared. I explained that this group includes specific genetic markers—DAO, HNMT, and AOC1—that play a significant role in histamine processing and immune responses.[143,144,145] For Chioma, this meant her body had a tendency to accumulate histamine, a compound involved in immune response, which could lead to inflammation, fatigue, and weight retention.

Chioma's eyes widened, visibly relieved but curious. "Histamine? Isn't that what antihistamines are for?"

"Yes, exactly," I explained. "Histamine isn't just about seasonal allergies. It's also naturally found in many foods, especially aged and fermented foods. For someone with your genetic profile, consuming these foods can lead to chronic inflammation, which explains the bloating, mood swings, and fatigue you've been experiencing."

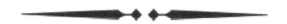

Science Spotlight

What is Histamine?

Histamine is a natural chemical in the body with key roles in immunity, digestion, and brain function. It is stored in cells like mast cells and released during immune responses, such as allergies, causing inflammation to fight off invaders.

Immune Response: Histamine causes symptoms like itching and swelling during allergic reactions.

Digestion: It stimulates stomach-acid production for digestion.

Brain Function: Acts as a neurotransmitter, influencing alertness and appetite.

When histamine isn't broken down effectively—due to genetics, enzyme deficiencies like DAO, or diet—it can build up, leading to symptoms like headaches, bloating, and fatigue.

Antihistamines block histamines' effects, offering relief for allergies or acid-related issues. However, addressing the root cause, such as histamine intolerance, requires a more tailored approach.

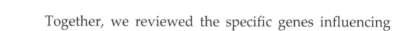

Together, we reviewed the specific genes influencing her symptoms:

- **DAO (diamine oxidase):** This enzyme breaks down histamine in the gut. Reduced DAO activity can lead to histamine overload and symptoms like bloating, migraines, and fatigue after eating high-histamine foods, such as smoked fish.[146]

- **HNMT (histamine n-methyltransferase):** This gene is crucial for histamine breakdown in the brain. Lower activity can impact mood stability and cognitive clarity, leading to mood swings and mental fog.[147]

- **AOC1 (amine oxidase copper-containing 1):** This gene supports histamine breakdown and detoxification. Reduced activity can lead to histamine buildup, exacerbating inflammation and discomfort.[148]

Why previous approaches didn't work based on these SNPs:

- **Intense exercise:** High-intensity workouts can increase cortisol and inflammatory markers, worsening symptoms for those with histamine intolerance due to DAO and AOC1 variations.[149]

- **Restrictive diets without focus on histamine:** Cutting calories or certain food groups without addressing high-histamine foods doesn't reduce histamine levels, leaving inflammation unchecked.[150]

- **Generic supplements:** Over-the-counter weight loss pills may contain stimulants or additives that increase histamine release, exacerbating symptoms for individuals with **HNMT** variations.[151]

As we went through her profile, Chioma shared that her favorite comfort food, jollof rice with smoked fish, was a staple in her diet. Unfortunately, the smoked fish was high in histamines, making it one of the culprits behind her persistent inflammation and discomfort. We discussed alternatives, like using fresh fish or baked chicken, to retain the dish's flavors without worsening her symptoms.

"But what about my workouts?" she asked. "I've been working out intensely for months, and it's not helping."

"Actually," I began, "intense workouts can elevate cortisol and increase inflammation, especially for those with an inflammatory profile like yours. Over-exercising can create a cycle where your body holds onto weight as a stress response rather than releasing it."[152]

For Chioma, these insights were transformative. She wasn't failing—she'd simply been working against her own biology. Now armed with knowledge about her genetic profile, Chioma finally felt hopeful and ready to make a change.

Phase Three: Personalized Steps for The Inflammatory Overload™

Working with women with The Inflammatory Overload™ necessitates a holistic plan to reduce inflammation, balance histamine levels, and align a fitness approach with their genetic needs. This transformation plan is about no longer about pushing harder, but working smarter with your body's natural tendencies.

1. GeneLean360° Tailored Nutrition Plan

Chioma's plan was built around foods that would help manage inflammation, support immune health, and nourish her in a way that aligned with her cultural preferences.

What Chioma tried before and why it didn't work:

- **Restrictive dieting (kale salads and deprivation):** Chioma tried to cut calories drastically by eating only salads.

  o **Why it didn't work:** While kale is nutritious, a restrictive diet can lack diversity and essential nutrients needed to reduce inflammation. Without addressing high-histamine foods, symptoms persisted.[153]

- **High-histamine foods in cultural dishes:** Her beloved smoked fish and fermented foods remained in her diet.

  o **Why it didn't work:** These foods are high in histamine, which can exacerbate inflammation in individuals with DAO and AOC1 variations.[154]

- **Skipping meals or inconsistent eating patterns:**

  o **Why it didn't work:** Irregular eating can stress the body, leading to cortisol release and increased inflammation, counteracting weight loss efforts.[155]

What worked instead:

- **Focus on low-histamine, anti-inflammatory foods:**

  o **Moderate protein:** Lean proteins like chicken, turkey, eggs, plant-based proteins like legumes and salmon, as well as fresh fish alternatives for her jollof rice.

Why: Protein stabilizes energy and helps prevent blood sugar spikes that can trigger histamine release and inflammation.[156]

- Healthy fats: Omega-3-rich foods such as salmon and chia seeds, along with avocado and olive oil.

- Omega-3 fatty acids: Salmon, chia seeds, flaxseeds.

- Monounsaturated fats: Avocado, olive oil.

Why: Omega-3s have anti-inflammatory properties, supporting cardiovascular health and reducing symptoms associated with inflammation.[157]

- Low to moderate carbohydrates: Complex carbs like quinoa, plantains, and yams.

Why: These complex carbs offer steady energy and support gut health without triggering insulin spikes, which can cascade into triggering an inflammatory responses.[158]

- **Histamine-lowering and anti-inflammatory foods:**

  - Fresh vegetables like cucumbers, zucchini, bell peppers, carrots.

Why: Low-histamine veggies add nutrients and fiber without increasing histamine load.[159]

- **Quercetin-rich foods:** Onions, apples, and broccoli.

Why: Quercetin acts as a natural antihistamine, helping to reduce inflammation and histamine sensitivity.[160]

2. GeneLean360° Targeted Supplementation™

Chioma's supplement protocol included HistAssist360°, designed to address her genetic predisposition to inflammation.

Key components

1. **Quercetin**

   o **Benefit:** This acts as a natural antihistamine and anti-inflammatory agent, stabilizing mast cells to prevent histamine release.[161]

   o **Why generic supplements didn't work:** Over-the-counter antihistamines don't provide the anti-inflammatory benefits of quercetin and may cause drowsiness or other side effects.

2. **Stinging nettle leaf**

   o **Benefit:** Stinging nettle supports immune function and reduces inflammation, helping to alleviate symptoms of histamine intolerance.[162]

   o **Why this works:** Nettle inhibits pro-inflammatory pathways, providing relief without the side effects of standard antihistamines.

3. **Bromelain**

   o **Benefit:** An enzyme from pineapple that aids digestion and reduces inflammation.[163]

   o **Why this works:** Improved digestion helps reduce the burden on the gut, where histamine is processed, and decreases systemic inflammation.

4. **N-acetyl cysteine (NAC)**

   o **Benefit:** This supports detoxification pathways, enhances glutathione production, and reduces oxidative stress.[164]

   o **Why this works:** By boosting glutathione levels, NAC aids in the breakdown of excess histamine and supports liver function.

5. **Vitamin C**

   o **Benefit:** Vitamin C helps degrade histamine and supports immune health.[165]

   o **Why generic supplements didn't work:** Standard vitamin C doses may not be sufficient to impact histamine levels significantly.

Why this targeted approach works:

- **Addresses genetic variations directly:** By focusing on nutrients that support histamine degradation and reduce inflammation, Chioma's supplementation protocol tackled the root causes of her symptoms.

- **Enhances detoxification pathways:** Supporting the body's natural detox systems helps eliminate excess histamine and reduce oxidative stress.

- **Reduces inflammation and supports immune function:** This comprehensive approach improved

Chioma's overall health, energy levels, and ability to lose weight.

3. GeneLean360° Personalized Fitness Plan

What Chioma tried before and why it didn't work:

- **Intense high-impact workouts:** High-intensity exercises can increase cortisol and inflammatory markers, counterproductive for those with inflammation-related genetic variations.[166]

- **Overtraining without adequate recovery:** Lack of recovery time exacerbates inflammation and fatigue, hindering progress and increasing injury risk.[167]

What worked instead:

- **Low-impact cardio for steady energy:**
  - **Frequency:** 3-4 days per week.
  - **Activities:** Walking, gentle cycling, and swimming.
  - **Duration:** 30-45 minutes per session.

Why: Low-impact cardio helped her stay active, balancing cardiovascular health without increasing cortisol or inflammation.[168]

- **Strength training for metabolic support:**
  - **Frequency:** 2-3 times per week.
  - **Focus:** Controlled, full-body exercises with lighter weights (e.g., lunges, squats, rows).
  - **Reps/sets:** 2-3 sets of 10-12 reps.

Why: Strength training helped Chioma build lean muscle mass, supporting a healthy metabolism without triggering cortisol spikes.[169]

- **Mind-body practices for relaxation:**
  - **Frequency:** 2-3 times per week.
  - **Activities:** Yoga, stretching, and deep breathing for 20-30 minutes.

Why: Mind-body exercises reduced cortisol, relaxed her nervous system, and helped her focus on healing rather than pushing through intense routines.[170]

- **Active recovery and rest days:**
  - **Frequency:** 1-2 rest days per week.
  - **Activities:** Light stretching, foam rolling, leisurely walks.
  - **Why:** Promotes muscle recovery and reduces inflammation, essential for overall progress.[171]

Why this works:

By shifting to a fitness routine that emphasizes gentle, consistent movement and adequate recovery, Chioma was able to stay active without triggering inflammation. This approach supported her weight loss goals while improving energy levels and reducing fatigue.

Chioma's Transformation and Breakthrough

Within weeks of following her new plan, Chioma noticed profound changes. Her energy became more stable, and she felt less bloated and inflamed. She found joy in her workouts again, relieved from the pressure of over-exerting herself. Over four months, Chioma shed *eighteen pounds* and came off her blood pressure medications, but more importantly, she felt lighter and healthier from within.

Chioma's journey wasn't just about losing weight—it was about reconnecting with her roots and embracing her body's needs. Through GeneLean360°'s The Inflammatory Overload™ approach, Chioma reclaimed her health, culture, and self-confidence.

■ *Lean Genes Blueprint* **Entry: Exploring Your Inflammation Triggers**

❖ Consider any signs of inflammation you've experienced—whether it's bloating, fatigue, or mood swings.

❖ Reflect on past diets or routines that may have worsened or improved these symptoms.

❖ Write down your thoughts on how a plan suited to your inflammatory responses could transform your results.

Chapter 13

The Sugar Shapers™

Sasha's story shows that sometimes the weight loss journey isn't about cutting carbs entirely—it's about finding the right balance for your unique metabolism. For The Sugar Shapers™, who struggle with insulin sensitivity and blood sugar stability, understanding these genetic factors is key to long-term success. With a personalized approach, Sasha was able to lose *sixty pounds* sustainably, stabilize her blood sugar, and finally feel energized. This chapter dives into how you, like Sasha, can transform cravings and energy swings into lasting health and balance

Have you ever felt that carbs are your enemy? Meet Sasha, a woman who once believed the only path to weight loss was cutting carbs altogether, enduring cravings, energy crashes, and a lingering frustration with her body. This chapter explores how her journey as one of The Sugar Shapers™ helped her overcome these struggles and transform her approach to health and weight loss.

Phase One: Understanding Sasha's Story

Sasha stood in front of her mirror, tugging at the dress she had hoped to wear for her upcoming wedding. The reflection staring back at her was not what she had envisioned for her special day. Desperate to lose fifty pounds before the wedding, she felt time slipping away. Traditional diets and grueling exercise routines had yielded minimal results, leaving her frustrated and anxious.

In a moment of desperation, Sasha turned to semaglutide injections, a medication gaining popularity for weight loss. Friends had raved about its effectiveness, and despite her reservations, she decided to try it. Initially, the pounds began to shed — five pounds the first week, then another fifteen over the next few months. She was elated, thinking she had found her miracle solution.

However, as weeks turned into months, Sasha began experiencing severe side effects. She felt constantly nauseous, suffered from debilitating stomach pains, and her energy levels plummeted. Despite losing twenty pounds, she felt worse than ever. After stopping the medication due to these side effects, not only did she regain the lost weight, but she also gained an additional ten pounds To make matters worse, she ended up in the hospital with gallbladder issues that required surgery — a complication associated with rapid weight loss and certain medications.[172]

Recovering at home, feeling defeated and scared, Sasha stumbled upon a free virtual event I was hosting about women's health and weight management. Intrigued by the idea of a personalized approach, she decided to attend. During the event, I discussed the importance of understanding one's genetic blueprint to achieve sustainable weight loss and overall health. I emphasized that weight struggles are often tied to genetic factors affecting metabolism, insulin sensitivity, and hormone balance.

Sasha was intrigued, but more than that, her fears subsided. She realized she wasn't broken and immune to losing weight, but rather her struggles could be a mismatch between conventional weight loss methods and her unique genetic makeup. Determined to find a lasting solution, she reached out to me for a consultation.

Phase Two: Discovering Sasha's Genetic Blueprint

In our initial meeting, Sasha shared her story—the highs of initial weight loss, the lows of severe side effects, and the frustration of regaining the weight. We discussed her diet, exercise routines, cravings, and energy levels throughout the day. I suggested genetic testing to gain insights into her body's unique needs.

When the results arrived, they revealed that Sasha belonged to a group we identify as The Sugar Shapers™. This group has specific genetic markers—TCF7L2, SLC30A8, and INSR genes—that significantly impact carbohydrate metabolism and insulin sensitivity.

- TCF7L2 (transcription factor 7-like 2): Variations in this gene are strongly associated with an increased risk of type 2 diabetes and affect insulin secretion and glucose production in the liver.[173] This explained Sasha's tendency for blood sugar spikes and crashes, leading to intense carbohydrate cravings.

- SLC30A8 (solute carrier family 30 member 8): This gene plays a crucial role in insulin granule function within pancreatic beta cells.[174] Variants can impair insulin secretion, contributing to poor blood sugar control after carbohydrate intake.

- INSR (insulin receptor gene): Mutations here can lead to insulin resistance, where cells do not respond effectively to insulin.[175] This resistance forces the body to produce more insulin to achieve glucose uptake, often leading to weight gain and difficulty losing weight.

Why previous approaches didn't work based on these SNPs:

- **Cutting carbs completely:** Going carb-free without addressing insulin sensitivity and blood sugar stability can lead to nutrient deficiencies and intense cravings, ultimately making the diet unsustainable.

- **Overreliance on medications like semaglutide:** While semaglutide can aid weight loss, it doesn't address genetic insulin resistance. Side effects like gastrointestinal discomfort are common, and for those with certain genetic predispositions, the medication may not provide sustainable results.[176]

- **Intense, high-impact exercise:** Intense workouts without proper fueling can lead to energy crashes and increased cortisol, further impairing insulin sensitivity.[177]

Understanding these genetic factors illuminated why standard diets and even medications hadn't provided Sasha with sustainable results. Her body was genetically predisposed to struggle with carbohydrate metabolism, making her susceptible to weight gain, energy crashes, and cravings when consuming a typical diet.

Sasha felt a mix of relief and frustration—relief in knowing there was a scientific explanation for her struggles, and frustration that she hadn't discovered this sooner. Armed with this new knowledge, she was eager to embark on a personalized plan tailored to her genetic profile.

Phase Three: Personalized Steps for The Sugar Shapers™

Equipped with insights from her genetic testing, I designed a comprehensive plan tailored to her unique metabolism. The focus was balanced nutrition, supplementation, and fitness strategies that worked with her genetics, not against them.

1. GeneLean360° Tailored Nutrition Plan

What Sasha had tried before and why it didn't work:

Strict low-carb diets: Sasha initially attempted carb elimination, thinking this would help her lose weight faster.

o **Why it didn't work:** Without balanced carbs, she experienced cravings, mood swings, and low energy. Her genetics indicated she needed the right type and portion of carbs to avoid blood sugar crashes.

Frequent, high-sugar snacks: In the past, Sasha had relied on snacks like granola bars and fruit juices for quick energy boosts.

- o **Why it didn't work:** High-sugar snacks led to blood sugar spikes followed by crashes, intensifying cravings and energy lulls.

- **Traditional low-calorie diets:**

  - o **Why it didn't work:** These diets didn't focus on the quality of carbohydrates or their glycemic impact, leading to blood sugar spikes and crashes. For someone with impaired insulin secretion and action, this can exacerbate weight gain and cravings.[178]

- **Skipping meals or extreme calorie restriction:**

  - o **Why it didn't work:** Irregular eating patterns can lead to hypoglycemia, triggering overeating and further destabilizing blood sugar levels.[179]

What worked instead:

- **Avoiding simple sugars:**

Sasha transitioned to consuming low-glycemic carbohydrates such as sweet potatoes, quinoa, and legumes. She avoided simple sugars and refined carbs found in white bread, pastries, and sugary snacks.

Just to clarify, this wasn't about a strict low-carb diet. Sasha's genetics showed she could still enjoy the carbs she loved—like sweet potatoes—without deprivation. We simply limited her carb portions to about one-quarter of her plate, ensuring that each serving was rich in fiber to slow glucose absorption.[180] This helped prevent rapid spikes in blood-sugar levels post-meals.

This approach kept her feeling satisfied and balanced, helping her avoid the blood sugar dips and cravings that could lead to overeating binges.

Why this approach works: High-fiber, complex carbs release glucose slowly into the bloodstream, which is crucial for individuals with TCF7L2 and SLC30A8 variants that impair insulin secretion and action.[181]

High protein and moderate healthy fats:

- **Lean proteins:** Each meal included sources like chicken breast, fish, turkey, eggs, tofu, or Greek yogurt. Protein helps slow gastric emptying, reducing the glycemic response of meals.[182]

- **Healthy fats:** Incorporation of monounsaturated fats from avocados, nuts, seeds, and olive oil provided satiety and further slowed carbohydrate absorption.

Why this approach works: As well as slowing gastric emptying, protein and healthy fats slow carbohydrate absorption, stabilizing blood sugar levels and enhancing satiety.[183,184] This is beneficial for those with INSR gene variations impacting insulin receptor function.[185]

Balanced meal timing with emphasis on breakfast:

- **Breakfast focus:** Sasha started her day with protein and fiber-rich breakfasts—like eggs with spinach and avocado or Greek yogurt with berries and chia seeds—to kickstart her metabolism and stabilize morning blood sugar levels.

- **Frequent smaller meals:** She ate every 3-4 hours, incorporating balanced snacks such as almond butter with apple slices or a handful of nuts with a piece of cheese.

Why this approach works: Regular meal timing prevents prolonged periods of low blood sugar, which can trigger overeating and cravings.[186] A substantial, balanced breakfast kickstarts metabolism and improves glycemic control throughout the day.[187]

2. GeneLean360° Targeted Supplementation™

We incorporated GlucoSupport360° into her daily routine—a supplement specifically designed for The Sugar Shapers™, targeting the genetic pathways affecting glucose metabolism.

Key ingredients:

- **Berberine:** Known to lower blood glucose levels by enhancing insulin sensitivity and promoting glycolysis, which helps break down sugars inside cells. Berberine also decreases glucose production in the liver.[188]

- **Cinnamon extract:** Cinnamon has been shown to improve insulin sensitivity and lower fasting blood glucose levels.[189] Cinnamon directly impacts pathways affected by SLC30A8 **and** TCF7L2 variants, aiding insulin secretion and action.

  o SLC30A8 variant (ZnT8 protein): The SLC30A8 gene encodes the ZnT8 protein, a zinc transporter critical for insulin storage and

147

release in pancreatic beta cells. Variants in SLC30A8 can impair zinc transport, weakening insulin secretion. Cinnamon enhances zinc bioavailability, which supports ZnT8 function, helping stabilize insulin storage and release even with this genetic impairment.[190,191]

○ TCF7L2 variant (GLP-1 pathway): TCF7L2 variants can reduce GLP-1 hormone activity, leading to lower insulin secretion. Cinnamon activates GLP-1 pathways, promoting insulin release and improving sensitivity, effectively compensating for TCF7L2-related insulin regulation issues.[192,193]

▪ **Chromium:** An essential trace mineral that enhances the action of insulin. Chromium improves glucose tolerance by increasing insulin receptor activity, beneficial for those with INSR gene variants.[194]

▪ **Alpha-lipoic acid (ALA):** A potent antioxidant that reduces oxidative stress and improves insulin sensitivity.[195] ALA enhances glucose uptake in muscle cells and reduces insulin resistance.

Why this targeted approach works:

▪ **Synergistic effects:** The combination of these ingredients addresses multiple aspects of glucose metabolism, from enhancing insulin sensitivity to reducing hepatic glucose production.

▪ **Genetic alignment:** The supplement targets the specific pathways affected by Sasha's genetic variants, offering a personalized approach to managing her blood sugar levels.

Cinnamon-rich foods:

In addition to the supplement, Sasha included cinnamon in her diet—adding it to smoothies, and incorporating it into baking.

3. GeneLean360° Personalized Fitness Plan

What Sasha tried before and why it didn't work:

- **Grueling exercise routines:** Many women feel they need to spend hours in the gym with intense, non-stop exercise to lose weight, which can lead to excessive fatigue and increased risk of injury. Without proper nutrition, these prolonged, high-intensity workouts can also elevate cortisol levels, impair insulin sensitivity, and cause energy crashes.[196]

- **Inconsistent exercise patterns:** Irregular exercise fails to deliver consistent metabolic benefits, which can hinder progress. Long workouts (45 minutes or more) can be mentally and physically exhausting, leading to burnout and inconsistency over time. Exercising intensely once a week doesn't match the results of a shorter, customized, and regular fitness plan.

- **Focus on cardio only:** Focusing solely on cardio overlooks muscle-building activities, which are essential for enhancing glucose uptake and improving insulin sensitivity.[197]

What worked:

▪ **Interval training**
   o **Frequency:** 2-3 times per week.

   o **Activities:** Sasha engaged in activities like sprint intervals on the treadmill, cycling bursts, or bodyweight circuits.

   o **Duration:** 20-30 minutes per session, with intervals of high-intensity effort followed by rest periods (e.g., 30 seconds of sprinting, 60 seconds of walking).

Why: Interval training burns calories efficiently and boosts metabolism long after the workout, improving insulin action and glucose metabolism. It's time-effective and adaptable, making it sustainable and reducing the risk of burnout.[198] It is also time-efficient, providing significant benefits in shorter time frames, fitting Sasha's busy schedule.

▪ **Strength training for lean muscle growth:**
   o **Frequency:** 2-3 times per week.

   o **Exercises:** Compound movements targeting large muscle groups—squats, deadlifts, lunges, bench presses, and rows.

   o **Reps/sets:** 3 sets of 8-12 reps with moderate to heavy weights.

Why: Strength training increases muscle mass. Muscle tissue is a major site for glucose disposal. Increasing muscle mass enhances basal metabolic rate and improves glucose uptake from the bloodstream.[199] Resistance training has also been shown to reduce insulin resistance, benefiting those with INSR gene variants.[200]

- **Steady-state cardio for recovery:**
  - o **Frequency:** 1-2 days per week.
  - o **Activities:** Brisk walking, light cycling, or swimming at a comfortable pace.
  - o **Duration:** 30-45 minutes per session.

Why: Steady-state cardio promotes fat oxidation, helps in burning fat without stressing the body, aiding weight loss. It also aids recovery, supports cardiovascular health and active recovery without increasing cortisol levels, which can negatively impact blood sugar.[201]

- **Mindfulness practices for stress reduction:**
  - o **Frequency:** 2-3 times per week.
  - o **Activities:** Meditation, deep-breathing exercises, or yoga for 15-20 minutes.

Why: Mindfulness reduces cortisol levels. High stress increases cortisol, which can raise blood sugar levels.[202] Mindfulness also improves insulin sensitivity. Stress management techniques have been shown to enhance insulin sensitivity and glucose control.[203]

Sasha's Transformation and Breakthrough

Over the next six months, Sasha embraced her personalized plan with determination, and the transformation was remarkable. Her weight steadily dropped, eventually reaching a total loss of *sixty pounds*—surpassing her initial goal. The changes were sustainable, with the majority of her weight loss coming from fat reduction, creating a visible improvement in her body composition and overall health.

As she continued to monitor her progress, Sasha found her blood-sugar levels stabilized within a healthy range, a change that alleviated the energy crashes and intense carb cravings that had once held her back. With each passing day, her energy levels increased, fueling her focus and lifting her mood. Sasha felt mentally sharp and emotionally balanced, a welcome shift that touched every area of her life.

The impact of her dedication became clear in her medical results as well. Sasha was thrilled to learn that her HbA1c levels had returned to a healthy range, officially bringing her out of the prediabetic category. For the first time in years, her risk of developing type 2 diabetes was significantly reduced, and she could approach her future with newfound peace of mind.[204]

As Sasha walked down the aisle on her wedding day, she radiated confidence and joy. She had not only achieved her weight-loss goal but also gained a deeper understanding of her body's unique needs. With the knowledge and habits that she'd developed, Sasha was well-equipped to embrace a fulfilling marriage, prepare for a safe, healthy pregnancy, and look forward to a vibrant life as her best self. Her journey had transformed her health, self-image, and outlook on the future—readying her to be the strong, thriving woman she aspired to be for herself, her marriage, and her future family.

Sasha's journey underscores the transformative power of personalized health strategies. By understanding and working with her genetic blueprint, she overcame challenges that once seemed insurmountable.

If you resonate with Sasha's story—struggling with weight despite your best efforts, experiencing energy crashes, and battling carb cravings—it may be time to explore your own genetic profile.

Visit GeneLean360.com to begin your personalized journey toward lasting health and vitality.

▣ *Lean Genes Blueprint* Entry: Managing Blood Sugar and Building a Balanced Plate

❖ Take a moment to reflect on your relationship with carbs and the impact they have on your energy, mood, and cravings.

❖ Think about ways to balance your meals with the right portions of protein, healthy fats, and fiber-rich carbs that leave you feeling satisfied rather than deprived.

Chapter 14

The Hormone Havoc™

Lori's journey is a testament to rediscovering balance in the face of hormonal upheaval. For women like Lori, who fall into The Hormone Havoc™ profile, managing weight and moods through menopause can feel like an impossible battle. Once a dedicated runner, Lori found herself sidelined by fatigue, stubborn weight gain, and unpredictable emotions. Traditional advice only left her more frustrated—until she learned that her genes were at the heart of her challenges. By creating a plan aligned with her unique genetic blueprint, Lori transformed her experience. Over four months, she regained control, shedding twenty-two pounds and reclaiming her energy and confidence.

Have you ever felt that hormonal changes have turned your life upside down, and nothing seems to help? Meet Lori, a woman who discovered that understanding her genetic makeup with The Hormone Havoc™ was the key to regaining control over her body and life. In this chapter, you'll see how you, like Lori, can navigate hormonal changes with personalized strategies that work with your biology, not against it.

Phase One: Understanding Lori's Story

Lori sat in her car outside the gym, gripping the steering wheel tightly. She stared blankly ahead, the rain tapping a steady rhythm on the windshield. Tears blurred her vision as she fought the overwhelming urge to just drive away. At fifty-two, Lori felt like a stranger in her own body. Once an avid runner who relished the challenge of a good workout, she now struggled to muster the energy to step through the gym doors.

It wasn't just the fatigue. Over the past year, Lori had watched helplessly as her weight crept up—twenty pounds that seemed to settle stubbornly around her midsection. Her clothes didn't fit right, and every glance in the mirror felt like a confrontation with someone she didn't recognize. The mood swings were the worst part. One moment she was irritable and snapping at her husband over trivial things; the next, she was fighting back tears during a commercial on TV. Sleep had become elusive, with nights spent tossing and turning, her mind racing with worries about work deadlines and her teenage daughter's struggles at school.

"Is this just aging?" she wondered aloud, her voice barely above a whisper. Lori feared this was her new normal—a life marked by exhaustion, weight gain, and emotional turbulence. She missed feeling like herself—confident, energetic, and in control.

Her doctor had suggested it was perimenopause and offered hormone replacement therapy (HRT), but Lori was hesitant. She'd read about the risks and wasn't convinced it was the right path for her. Friends recommended various diets, supplements, and meditation apps. She tried them all—keto, IF, yoga—but nothing seemed to make a lasting difference. The weight wouldn't budge, her moods were still unpredictable, and the brain fog persisted.

One sleepless night, scrolling through her phone in the dark, Lori stumbled upon a webinar I was hosting about hormonal balance and genetics. The title caught her eye: "Unlocking Hormone Harmony Through Your Unique Genetic Blueprint." Skeptical yet desperate, she signed up.

Phase Two: Discovering Lori's Genetic Blueprint

When I first met Lori during our consultation, she was forthright about her struggles. "I feel like I'm falling apart," she confessed. "I don't recognize myself anymore, and it's terrifying."

I listened attentively as she described her symptoms— weight gain, fatigue, mood swings, insomnia—and her frustrations with the lack of lasting solutions. I assured her she wasn't alone and that many women experience similar challenges during perimenopause and menopause.

"We have the option to look deeper," I suggested. "Genetic testing can provide insights into how your body is uniquely processing hormonal changes."

Lori agreed, hopeful this might finally offer some answers.

When her results came in, we sat down together to interpret them. "Lori," I began, "your genetic profile places you in a group we call The Hormone Havoc™. You have specific variations in the ESR1, ESR2, and CYP19A1 genes."

Intrigued but cautious, she asked, "What does that mean for me?"

"Let's break it down," I said.

- **ESR1 and ESR2 (estrogen receptor 1 and 2):**

  o **Role:** These genes encode the receptors that estrogen binds to in the body.

  o **Variation impact:** Variations can alter how sensitive your tissues are to estrogen fluctuations.[205] For you, this means the natural decline in estrogen during perimenopause is causing more pronounced symptoms—like mood swings, hot flashes, and weight gain—compared to others without these variations.

- **CYP19A1 (cytochrome P450 family 19 subfamily A member 1):**

  o **Role:** This gene is responsible for encoding aromatase, an enzyme that converts androgens into estrogen.

  o **Variation impact:** Variations can affect estrogen synthesis, potentially leading to imbalances that exacerbate menopausal symptoms.[206]

Why previous approaches didn't work based on these SNPs:

- **HRT:** Without knowing her genetic variations, HRT might not effectively balance her hormones and could increase the risk of adverse effects.[207] Variations in CYP19A1 can influence how her body metabolizes hormones, affecting HRT efficacy.

- **Generic diets:** Diets like keto may not provide sufficient phytoestrogens or support estrogen metabolism, failing to address the issues caused by ESR1 and ESR2 variations.[208]

- **Intense exercise:** High cortisol from intense workouts can worsen hormonal imbalances, especially in those with estrogen receptor sensitivities.[209]

- **Over-the-counter supplements:** Generic supplements don't target the specific genetic pathways affected in Lori's case, such as estrogen receptor function and aromatase activity.[210]

- **Meditation and yoga alone:** While helpful for stress reduction, they don't directly influence estrogen metabolism affected by her genetic variations.

Lori's eyes welled up. "So, it's not all in my head?"

"Not at all," I assured her. "Your genes are influencing how your body responds to hormonal changes. The good news is that we can create a personalized plan to support your body through this transition."

Relief washed over her face. "Where do we start?"

Phase Three: Personalized Steps for The Hormone Havoc™

Understanding Lori's genetic predispositions allowed us to tailor a comprehensive plan addressing her unique hormonal needs.

1. GeneLean360° Tailored Nutrition Plan

What Lori tried before and why it didn't work:

Ketogenic diet:

o **Why it didn't work:** The keto diet is low in carbohydrates and can reduce intake of phytoestrogens and fiber, which are crucial for estrogen metabolism and balance.[211]

Intermittent fasting:

o **Why it didn't work:** IF can increase cortisol levels and stress on the body, potentially worsening hormonal imbalances and mood swings in menopausal women.[212]

Calorie restriction:

o **Why it didn't work:** Severe calorie restriction can lead to nutrient deficiencies, impairing hormone production and exacerbating fatigue.[213]

What worked instead:

▪ **Hormone-balancing foods:**

o **Phytoestrogen-rich foods,** including Flaxseeds, soybeans, lentils, and chickpeas.

Why this works: Phytoestrogens can bind to estrogen receptors, providing mild estrogenic effects that help alleviate symptoms caused by declining estrogen levels.[214] This is especially beneficial for those with ESR1 and ESR2 variations affecting estrogen receptor sensitivity.

- o **Cruciferous vegetables,** including broccoli, Brussels sprouts, and kale.

Why this works: These contain indole-3-carbinol, which supports estrogen metabolism and helps balance hormone levels.[215]

- **Macronutrient balance**
  - o **Lean proteins,** Including fish rich in omega-3 fatty acids (salmon, mackerel), chicken, turkey, and plant-based proteins like quinoa.

Why this works: Protein supports muscle mass maintenance, which is crucial as estrogen decline can lead to decreased muscle and increased fat mass.[216] Omega-3s also have anti-inflammatory properties and can improve mood.[217]

  - o **Healthy fats,** including avocados, nuts (especially walnuts and almonds), seeds (flaxseeds, chia seeds), and olive oil.

Why this works: Healthy fats are essential for hormone production and can help reduce inflammation.[218] They also promote satiety, reducing overeating.

  - o **Complex carbohydrates:**

    Inclusion: Quinoa, chia seeds and legumes.

    Why this works: High in fiber, these carbs stabilize blood sugar levels, preventing energy crashes and mood swings.[219]

- **Meal timing and mindful eating:**

  o **Balanced breakfasts,** starting the day with protein and fiber, such as a veggie omelet with spinach and wholegrain toast.

Why this works: Helps maintain stable blood sugar throughout the day, reducing cravings and supporting energy levels.[220]

  o **Mindful eating practices:** Encouraging Lori to eat slowly, savor her food, and listen to her body's hunger and fullness cues.

Why this works: Reduces overeating and improves digestion, which can be affected by hormonal changes.[221]

2. GeneLean360° Targeted Supplementation™

Lori's personalized supplementation plan tailored to her genetic profile, included Fembalance360° directly addressing her hormonal imbalances.

- **Key ingredient:** Rhapontic rhubarb root extract (ERr 731)

- **Mechanism of action:**

  o **Selective estrogen receptor modulator (SERM):** ERr 731 selectively binds to estrogen receptors, providing estrogen-like benefits without the risks associated with traditional HRT.[222]

  o **Symptom relief:** Clinical studies have shown significant reductions in menopausal symptoms, including hot flashes, mood swings, and sleep disturbances.[223]

Additional supplements:

- **Vitamin D:**
  - **Benefit:** Essential for bone health, which becomes a concern during menopause due to decreased estrogen levels.[224]

Why this works: Supports calcium absorption and bone mineralization, countering the effects of estrogen decline influenced by genetic variations.

- **Magnesium:**
  - **Benefit:** Supports sleep quality, muscle relaxation, and mood stabilization.[225]

Why this works: Helps mitigate symptoms of fatigue and insomnia, addressing issues not resolved by previous supplements.

- **B-complex vitamins:**
  - **Benefit:** Aid in energy production, cognitive function, and reducing symptoms of depression and anxiety.[226]

Why this works: Supports overall neurological function and mood, which can be affected by hormonal fluctuations and genetic predispositions.

3. GeneLean360° Personalized Fitness Plan

What Lori tried before and why it didn't work:

- **Intense running and high-intensity workouts:** These activities can increase cortisol levels, leading to further hormonal imbalance, fatigue, and weight gain around the midsection.[227]

- **Yoga and meditation alone:** While helpful for stress reduction, they didn't provide the strength training needed to counteract muscle loss due to decreased estrogen.

What worked instead:

- **Strength training for muscle maintenance**:
  o **Frequency:** 3 times per week.

  o **Exercises:** Resistance training focusing on major muscle groups—squats, lunges, chest presses, and rows.

  o **Why:** Helps counteract the loss of muscle mass due to decreased estrogen, boosts metabolism, and supports bone density.[228]

- **Cardiovascular exercise for heart health:**
  o **Frequency:** 3-4 times per week.

  o **Activities:** Brisk walking, cycling, swimming.

  o **Why:** Improves cardiovascular health without excessively raising cortisol levels[21]. Supports heart health, which is crucial as the risk of heart disease increases post-menopause.

- **Mind-body practices for stress reduction**:
  o **Frequency:** Daily, even if just for 10 minutes.

  o **Activities:** Yoga, tai chi, or meditation.

  o **Why:** Reduces cortisol levels, alleviates stress, and improves sleep quality.[229] High cortisol can exacerbate hormonal imbalances and weight gain, particularly around the abdomen.

- **Active recovery and rest:**
  - **Importance:** Ensures adequate recovery time to prevent overtraining and additional stress on the body.
  - **Why this works:** Supports hormonal balance by preventing cortisol spikes and allowing the body to repair and rebuild.

Lori's Transformation and Breakthrough

Within a month of implementing her personalized plan, Lori began noticing subtle changes. Her energy levels improved, and she no longer needed multiple cups of coffee to get through the day. The brain fog started to lift, and she found it easier to focus at work.

After six weeks, Lori had lost *ten pounds*—not just on the scale, but she felt it in the way her clothes fit and the return of muscle tone. Her mood swings became less frequent and less intense. "I had a disagreement with my daughter the other day," she shared during a follow-up session. "But instead of snapping, I was able to stay calm and actually listen to her."

By four months, Lori felt like a new person. She had lost a total of *twenty-two pounds*, but more importantly, she regained confidence in her body and mind. Her sleep improved significantly; she was getting seven to eight hours of restful sleep most nights. The hot flashes and night sweats had diminished drastically.

"I can't believe the difference," she told me, her eyes shining. "I feel like myself again. Actually, I feel better than I have in years."

Lori's journey illustrates the profound impact that understanding one's genetic makeup can have on navigating hormonal changes. By addressing her unique genetic profile, we were able to tailor interventions that alleviated her symptoms and improved her overall quality of life.

If you find yourself resonating with Lori's experience—struggling with unexplained weight gain, mood swings, fatigue, and other menopausal symptoms—consider exploring your own genetic blueprint.

Remember, menopause is a natural transition, but it doesn't have to diminish your quality of life. With personalized strategies, you can embrace this new chapter with vitality and confidence.

◼ *Lean Genes Blueprint* Entry: Reflecting on Your Hormonal Balance Journey

Reflect on your own experiences with hormonal shifts and their impact on your life. Think about how these changes have influenced your mood, energy, and overall wellness.

❖ What solutions have you tried in the past?

❖ Were they effective?

❖ Consider what a customized, hormone-supportive approach could look like for you.

If you're struggling with hot flashes, mood swings, stubborn weight gain, or low energy, I created Fembalance360° for you. This four-week system includes comprehensive videos and a planner to guide you through personalized strategies that help you regain hormonal balance and feel like yourself again.

Head to genelean360.com/store to learn more.

Chapter 15

The Detox Bound™

Chiara's journey shows how understanding your genetic blueprint can break through stubborn weight loss resistance. For The Detox Bound™, weight gain isn't about lack of effort. It's about a body overwhelmed by toxins due to genetic variations in detoxification pathways. By supporting her unique genetic needs, Chiara reclaimed her vitality and confidence. Through a personalized detoxification protocol, she lost fifteen pounds in three months, transforming not just her body but her entire sense of self. This chapter reveals how, like Chiara, you can unlock your body's natural detoxification power to achieve lasting weight loss.

Have you ever felt trapped in a body that doesn't feel like your own, despite your best efforts to lose weight and feel energized? Meet Chiara, a woman who discovered that understanding her genetic makeup as one of The Detox Bound™ was the key to unlocking her body's potential and achieving lasting change.

Phase One: Understanding Chiara's Story

Chiara stood in front of her closet, a familiar knot forming in her stomach. The dress she had planned to wear to her friend's wedding—a sleek, emerald-green number that once hugged her figure perfectly—now clung uncomfortably to her midsection. She tugged at the fabric, trying to smooth out the bulges that seemed to have appeared overnight. Her arms, once toned from hours at the gym, now felt soft, and she hated how they looked when they were exposed. With a sigh, she tossed the dress onto the growing pile of clothes that no longer fit and reached for something loose and forgiving.

At forty-two, Chiara felt trapped in a body she didn't recognize. Despite her best efforts—countless diets, intense workout regimens, and every detox cleanse she could find—her weight continued to creep up. The fatigue was relentless; even after ten hours of sleep, she woke up exhausted. Dark circles under her eyes had become a permanent fixture, and her once-radiant skin looked dull and lifeless.

Her self-esteem plummeted. Intimacy with her partner became a source of anxiety. She avoided his touch, fearing he'd notice the changes she couldn't ignore. "I just don't feel like myself," she confided in her sister one afternoon. "It's like I'm stuck in someone else's body, and no matter what I do, I can't get back to me."

Chiara tried to mask her insecurity with baggy clothes and a forced smile, but inside, she was desperate for a solution. The final straw came when, after months of rigorous exercise and strict dieting, she stepped on the scale to find she'd gained another five pounds Frustrated and heartbroken, she broke down in tears.

Scrolling through social media late one night, Chiara stumbled upon an article discussing how genetics could impact weight loss and detoxification. Intrigued, she clicked through to learn about a program called GeneLean360°, which focused on personalized health strategies based on your genetic makeup. She read stories of others who had struggled like her and found success through this approach.

With renewed hope, Chiara scheduled a consultation.

Phase Two: Discovering Chiara's Genetic Blueprint

When Chiara arrived at my office, she carried not just the weight of her body but the weight of her emotions.

"I've tried everything," she began, her voice quivering. "Low-carb, vegan, intermittent fasting. I work out until I'm exhausted, but the scale won't budge. I look in the mirror and hate what I see. I feel so... undesirable."

I leaned forward and replied, "Chiara, your struggle is real, and it's not your fault. Your body is sending signals that we need to understand."

We decided to delve deeper with genetic testing to uncover any underlying factors contributing to her weight loss resistance.

The results were illuminating. Chiara belonged to a group I call The Detox Bound™, characterized by specific genetic variations affecting detoxification processes:

- **CYP1A2:** This gene influences phase I liver detoxification, responsible for metabolizing toxins and hormones. Chiara's variation led to a sluggish phase I detox, causing toxins to accumulate in her system and contribute to fatigue and hormonal imbalances.[230]

- **GSTM1:** Essential for phase II detoxification, this gene helps neutralize toxins for elimination. Chiara had a GSTM1 deletion, reducing her body's ability to produce glutathione, a critical antioxidant for detoxification. This deficiency meant her body struggled to neutralize harmful compounds, leading to toxin buildup.[231]

- **NAT2:** This gene is involved in processing environmental toxins and certain medications. Chiara's variant classified her as a slow acetylator, meaning toxins lingered longer in her system, exacerbating her symptoms of fatigue and weight gain.[232]

Why previous approaches didn't work based on these SNPs:

- **Generic diets and exercise plans:** Standard diets and workouts don't address the accumulation of toxins due to impaired detox pathways. Without supporting detoxification, her body held onto weight as a protective mechanism.[233]

- **Over-the-counter detox cleanses:** These cleanses often stimulate phase I detoxification without supporting phase II, leading to increased circulating toxins that can cause further fatigue and oxidative stress.[234]

- **Generic supplements:** Supplements not tailored to her genetic needs failed to provide the necessary support for her detoxification pathways and may have added to her toxic burden.[235]

"Your body isn't failing you," I explained gently. "It's simply overwhelmed. These genetic factors are making it harder for your body to eliminate toxins, which can get trapped in fat cells. This isn't about willpower or effort; it's about giving your body the support it needs."

She stared at the test results, a mix of relief and frustration on her face. "So, all this time, I've been fighting my own body without knowing why?"

"Exactly," I affirmed. "But now that we understand what's happening, we can create a plan tailored to your unique needs."

To fully grasp Chiara's struggle, it's essential to understand the science behind how toxins impact weight management.

1. **Phase I and II liver detoxification:** The liver detoxifies harmful substances in two phases. In phase I, toxins are modified into intermediate forms, which can sometimes be more toxic. Phase II involves conjugating these intermediates with molecules like glutathione, making them water-soluble for excretion. When either phase is impaired—due to genetic variations like Chiara's—the detox process slows down, leading to toxin accumulation.[236]

2. **Toxins trapped in fat cells:** The body, in an attempt to protect vital organs, stores excess toxins in fat cells. This not only increases fat storage but also makes it difficult to lose weight, as releasing these toxins without proper support can overwhelm the body.[237]

3. **Hormonal disruption:** Toxins can mimic or interfere with hormones, affecting metabolism, appetite regulation, and fat storage. This hormonal imbalance contributes to weight gain and makes weight loss efforts less effective.[238]

4. **Inflammation and insulin resistance:** Accumulated toxins promote chronic inflammation, which can lead to insulin resistance—a key factor in weight gain and difficulty losing weight.[239]

Understanding this science provided Chiara with clarity. Her feelings of despair weren't a result of personal failure, but a complex interplay of genetics and biochemistry.

Phase Three: Personalized Steps for The Detox Bound™

With this knowledge, I crafted a comprehensive, personalized plan to support Chiara's detoxification pathways and address her weight loss resistance.

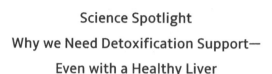

Science Spotlight

Why we Need Detoxification Support—

Even with a Healthy Liver

A common argument against detox supplements is that our bodies already have a liver, which functions as a natural detoxifier. While it's true that the liver is equipped with powerful detoxification systems, the modern environment exposes our bodies to unprecedented levels of toxins.

Here's why additional support can make a significant difference:

1. **Our toxic load has increased drastically:** The liver evolved to handle natural metabolic waste and occasional environmental toxins. Today, however, we're exposed to thousands of man-made chemicals daily— from pesticides and food additives to pollutants and plastics. This toxic load overtaxes the liver's natural capacity, causing toxins to accumulate over time.

2. **Detoxification happens in phases, and imbalances are common:** The liver's detox process is complex and involves two main phases. In phase I, enzymes break down toxins into reactive intermediates, which can be more harmful than the original toxin. Phase II then neutralizes these intermediates for safe elimination.[240] If either phase is sluggish (which can happen due to genetics or lifestyle factors), toxins build up and are stored in fat cells, leading to weight gain, fatigue, and inflammation.

3. **Nutrient demand for detoxification is high:** Each phase of detoxification requires specific nutrients to function optimally. For instance, glutathione is essential for phase II detoxification, but many people are low in this critical antioxidant due to stress, poor diet, or aging. Without adequate nutrient support, detox pathways

become inefficient, and the liver's ability to process and eliminate toxins is compromised.[241]

4. **Hormonal interference by toxins:** Many toxins, called endocrine disruptors, mimic or interfere with hormones, causing metabolic disruptions that contribute to weight gain and other health issues. The liver plays a major role in hormone balance by breaking down and clearing excess hormones, but when overloaded, these hormone-like toxins accumulate in the body, leading to hormone imbalances and metabolic resistance.[242]

5. **Genetic variations can slow detoxification:** Certain genetic variations can make some people less efficient at processing specific toxins. For example, variations in genes like CYP1A2 and GSTM1 can impact how quickly or effectively the liver detoxifies various substances. These individuals may benefit from targeted support to enhance their unique detox pathways.[243]

6. **Age and stress impact liver function:** Liver function naturally declines with age, and factors like stress, poor sleep, and a sedentary lifestyle can further impair detoxification. As the liver slows down, it becomes harder to keep up with toxin processing, making additional detox support increasingly valuable.[244]

In sum, while the liver is indeed a powerhouse, the high toxin load and nutrient demands of modern life make supplemental detox support a powerful tool for optimizing health. By strategically supporting the liver's natural functions, we can enhance its capacity to handle the toxins we encounter every day.

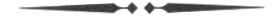

1. GeneLean360° Tailored Nutrition Plan

What Chiara tried before and why it didn't work:

Fad diets and cleanses:

- o **Why they didn't work:** These approaches often lack essential nutrients needed for detoxification and can stress the body further, impairing detox pathways.[245]

Calorie restriction:

- o **Why it didn't work:** Severely limiting calories can slow metabolism and reduce the body's ability to produce detoxification enzymes.[246]

What to try instead:

Foods to support detoxification:

Cruciferous vegetables:

- o **Inclusion:** Broccoli, kale, Brussels sprouts.

- o **Why:** Contain compounds that induce phase II detox enzymes, aiding in the conjugation and elimination of toxins.[247]

Sulfur-rich foods:

- o **Inclusion:** Garlic, onions, eggs.

- o **Why:** Provide building blocks for glutathione production, a key antioxidant in detoxification.[248]

Antioxidant-rich fruits:

- o **Inclusion:** Berries, citrus fruits.

o **Why:** Combat oxidative stress caused by toxin accumulation, supporting liver health.[249]

High-fiber foods:

o **Inclusion:** Lentils, chickpeas, whole grains.

o **Why:** Fiber binds to toxins in the gut, promoting their elimination and preventing reabsorption.[250]

Hydration:

o **Inclusion:** Increased water intake, adding lemon to support liver function.

o **Why:** Adequate hydration supports kidney function and helps flush out water-soluble toxins.[251]

Why this approach works:

By providing the nutrients necessary for both phase I and phase II detoxification, this nutrition plan directly supports Chiara's genetic detoxification challenges. It supplies the substrates needed for glutathione production and enhances the body's ability to neutralize and eliminate toxins.

2. GeneLean360° Targeted Supplementation™

I introduced targeted supplements to enhance her detox processes:

- **Restore360°**

   Purpose: Supports Phase II detoxification and Phase III elimination, crucial for Chiara's impaired detox pathways.

Key ingredients:

- N-acetylcysteine (NAC): It boosts glutathione production, aiding in detoxification of heavy metals and environmental toxins.[252]
- Glycine and taurine: These are essential amino acids for conjugation reactions in Phase II detoxification.[253]
- Antioxidants: Alpha-lipoic acid and green tea extract reduce oxidative stress caused by toxin buildup.[254]
- Fiber and protein: These support gut health and aid in toxin elimination through the digestive tract.[255]

CoreEnergy360°

Purpose: Provides essential vitamins and minerals to recharge cellular energy and support detox pathways.

Key ingredients:

- B vitamins (B6, B12, folate): Crucial for methylation processes in detoxification and energy production.[256]
- Alpha-lipoic acid and acetyl l-carnitine: These support mitochondrial function, enhancing energy levels and fat metabolism.[257]
- Antioxidants: Green tea extract, broccoli seed extract, and resveratrol protect mitochondria from oxidative damage.[258]

LiverComplete360°

Purpose: Stimulates phase I detoxification once phase II is underway, ensuring a balanced detox process.

Key ingredients:

- Silymarin (milk thistle): Milk thistle protects liver cells from toxin-induced damage and supports regeneration.[259]

- Artichoke extract and dandelion root: These promote bile production and flow, aiding in the digestion and elimination of fats and fat-soluble toxins.[260]

- Turmeric (curcumin): Turmeric reduces inflammation and oxidative stress in the liver.[261]

Implementation plan:

- **Days 1-2:** Start with Restore360° twice daily to activate phase II detox pathways, ensuring that toxins can be safely neutralized.

  - **Why this works when other detoxes do not:** Many "detoxes" focus on phase-I detoxification first, which can release reactive toxins that overwhelm the body, if phase II isn't ready to neutralize them. By starting with phase II, Restore360° safely prepares the body for toxin processing, avoiding the side effects of incomplete detoxification.[262,263]

- **Day 3 onward:** Add LiverComplete360° to stimulate phase I detoxification, now that Phase II is adequately supported.

  ○ **Why this works when other detoxes do not:** Other "detoxes" that jump into phase I alone can overburden the liver with too many active toxins at once. By introducing LiverComplete360° after phase II activation, this plan avoids flooding the body with toxins, creating a balanced detox that reduces stress on the liver and promotes safe elimination.[264,265]

- **Daily**: Take CoreEnergy360° to maintain energy levels and support overall detoxification.

  ○ **Why this works when other detoxes do not**: Many "detoxes" lack essential nutrients and lead to fatigue. CoreEnergy360° provides critical B vitamins, antioxidants, and amino acids to sustain energy and cellular function, so detoxing doesn't leave the body drained or undernourished.[266,267]

3. GeneLean360° Personalized Fitness Plan

What Chiara tried before and why it didn't work:

- **Intense workouts:** High-intensity exercises increased cortisol levels, leading to further hormonal imbalances and taxing her already overburdened detoxification system.[268]

What worked instead:

- **Low-impact cardio:** Walking and swimming to improve circulation and lymphatic flow, aiding in toxin elimination without stressing the body.[269]

- **Yoga and stretching:** To reduce stress hormones, support hormonal balance and enhances relaxation.[270]

- **Rebounding:** Gentle bouncing on a mini-trampoline to stimulate lymphatic drainage promoting detoxification.[271]

Why this approach works when everything else did not:

By focusing on gentle, restorative exercises, Chiara's fitness plan supports detoxification processes, reduces stress on the body, and avoids exacerbating cortisol levels, which can hinder weight loss.

4. Lifestyle Modifications

- **Sleep hygiene:** Establishing a regular sleep schedule to support hormonal regulation and recovery.[272,273]

- **Stress reduction:** Incorporating mindfulness and deep-breathing exercises to lower cortisol levels, which can impact weight and detoxification.[274,275]

Chiara's Transformation and Breakthrough

The changes didn't happen overnight, but within weeks, Chiara began to notice subtle improvements. Her energy levels increased, and the brain fog started to lift. "I woke up feeling refreshed for the first time in years," she shared enthusiastically.

By the third month, the scale finally reflected her efforts—a loss of *fifteen pounds*. More importantly, she felt alive. The chronic fatigue had faded, her skin glowed, and the dark circles under her eyes diminished. She rediscovered joy in activities she had long abandoned.

Her relationship with her partner blossomed. "I don't shy away from his touch anymore," she confided. "I feel desirable again, not just physically but emotionally. I'm reconnecting with myself."

Chiara's journey was a testament to the power of personalized health strategies. By understanding her genetic blueprint, she moved from despair to empowerment, reclaiming not just her body but her self-worth.

Her story resonates with many women who silently battle similar struggles—feeling trapped, undesirable, and hopeless despite their best efforts. If you find yourself relating to her journey, remember that you're not alone, and it's not a reflection of your effort or worth.

Exploring your genetic blueprint can unveil underlying factors contributing to weight loss resistance. By aligning your health strategies with your body's unique needs, you can break free from the cycle of despair and step into a life of vitality and self-love.

▣ *Lean Genes Blueprint* Entry: Reflecting on Your Detoxification Journey

Reflect on your experiences with weight loss resistance and fatigue.

- ❖ What solutions have you tried in the past?

- ❖ Were they effective?

- ❖ How could understanding your unique genetic detoxification pathways change your approach to health and weight management?

I created the 14-Day Restore360° System after noticing a significant pattern in the women I worked with. Many had deletions in their GSTM1 and CYP1A2 genes, impairing their natural detox pathways, and were experiencing persistent symptoms like fatigue, weight gain, and inflammation.

For these women, traditional methods simply weren't enough. On the 14-Day Restore360° System alone, we've seen women lose an average of ten to twelve pounds, reduce bloating, and regain their energy levels.

To find out how this system can help support your unique detox needs, visit genelean360.com/restore360

Chapter 16

The Vascular Vulnerables™

Lisa's story reveals how genetic predispositions can impact heart health and weight loss success. For The Vascular Vulnerables™, traditional diets often fall short because they don't address the underlying cardiovascular challenges that affect energy, stamina, and metabolism. Women like Lisa often feel betrayed by their bodies, watching their blood pressure and cholesterol rise despite their best efforts.

By supporting her unique genetic needs, Lisa transformed not just her numbers, but her entire life. She lost twenty-eight pounds over four months, while her blood pressure dropped from 142/90 to 118/75, and her cholesterol levels normalized. Within three months, she regained the energy to keep up with her kids—all while protecting her long-term heart health.

This chapter reveals how, like Lisa, you can optimize your cardiovascular health to achieve lasting vitality and confidence.

Have you ever felt your body wasn't responding the way it should, despite your best efforts, especially when it comes to heart health and weight loss? Meet Lisa, a woman who discovered that understanding her genetic makeup as one of The Vascular Vulnerables™ was the key to transforming her health and reclaiming her vitality.

Phase One: Understanding Lisa's Story

Lisa, a forty-five-year-old entrepreneur and mother of two, was the embodiment of dedication—whether in her business, family life, or health pursuits. Yet as the years passed, her health seemed to stall, hitting her with unexpected setbacks. Even after regular workouts and a heart-conscious diet, she found herself breathless after climbing stairs, fatigued after a day's work, and worrying about her rising blood pressure and cholesterol levels.

"I feel like my body is betraying me," she admitted during our first meeting. "I used to be able to run miles, keep up with my kids, and feel on top of my game. But now, I just feel... tired and out of shape."

Her family's medical history weighed heavily on her mind. Her parents had both suffered heart attacks in their early sixties, and her doctor had recently expressed concerns about her elevated LDL cholesterol. Despite being disciplined with her health routines, she felt like her body was slipping out of her control, and her confidence dwindled.

Phase Two: Discovering Lisa's Genetic Blueprint

After joining the GeneLean360° Genetic Gateway, we explored her family history and conducted a genetic test. Her results confirmed she was part of The Vascular Vulnerables™ group, with genetic variations in APOE, ACE, and LPA—indicating the need for a more precise cardiovascular support strategy. We designed a tailored plan to help her safeguard her heart health, optimize stamina, and bring lasting vitality back into her life.

The results of Lisa's genetic test revealed key insights into her unique cardiovascular needs:

- **APOE (apolipoprotein E):** This gene influences cholesterol transport and metabolism, affecting LDL cholesterol levels. Individuals with certain APOE variants (Lisa has the APOE ε4 variant) are predisposed to higher LDL cholesterol and triglyceride levels, increasing their risk for cardiovascular issues if not managed.[276]

- **ACE (angiotensin-converting enzyme):** ACE plays a significant role in regulating blood pressure. Lisa's ACE gene variant increased her susceptibility to elevated blood pressure, as well as decreased vascular flexibility, placing added strain on her cardiovascular system.[277]

- **LPA (lipoprotein(a)):** The LPA gene variant in Lisa's results indicated a tendency for elevated levels of lipoprotein(a), a type of LDL cholesterol linked to increased risk of atherosclerosis and cardiovascular disease.[278]

Why previous approaches didn't work based on these SNPs:

- **Generic diets:** Standard heart-healthy diets may not sufficiently lower LDL cholesterol or lipoprotein(a) levels in individuals with APOE ε4 and LPA variants.[279]

- **Standard exercise routines:** High-intensity workouts can elevate blood pressure and place additional strain on the cardiovascular system, which may be less effective or even counterproductive for individuals with certain ACE gene variations. People with the ACE I/I variant, for example, may respond better to endurance-focused, steady-state activities rather than high-intensity routines that emphasize power and strength.[280]

- **Generic supplements:** Over-the-counter omega-3s and multivitamins lack the potency and specific formulation needed to impact her genetic cardiovascular risks.[281]

- **Stress management alone:** While beneficial, these methods don't directly influence cholesterol metabolism or blood pressure regulation affected by her genetic variations.[282]

I explained to Lisa, "Your genetics are like a roadmap, highlighting areas that need extra support to keep your heart healthy and resilient. Knowing your genetic tendencies allows us to focus on protecting your cardiovascular health more effectively."

Lisa's eyes filled with relief. Finally, she had answers and could see a path forward beyond what typical diets and routines had provided.

For The Vascular Vulnerables™, understanding how cardiovascular health interacts with weight loss is essential. Here's how specific mechanisms impact individuals with Lisa's genetic profile.

- **Cholesterol metabolism and storage in arteries:** APOE and LPA gene variants can lead to inefficient cholesterol transport and higher levels of lipoprotein(a), which predispose individuals to LDL cholesterol accumulation. This buildup leads to arterial plaque formation, causing atherosclerosis and impairing blood flow, which can limit stamina and affect weight loss efforts.[283,284]

- **Blood pressure regulation:** With ACE gene variations, the body has a harder time managing blood pressure. This can result in higher blood pressure levels, placing more strain on the heart and vascular system. Over time, this stress contributes to arterial stiffness, making cardiovascular exercise and stamina maintenance more challenging.[285]

- **Inflammation and oxidative stress:** Elevated cholesterol levels and increased blood pressure contribute to inflammation and oxidative stress in the arteries, making them more vulnerable to damage. This inflammation not only increases cardiovascular risk, but also impairs the body's ability to metabolize fats efficiently, leading to greater weight retention.[286]

Understanding the genetic and biochemical layers in Lisa's case provided a clear path forward. The solution was not just about effort, but about aligning her plan with her body's specific cardiovascular needs.

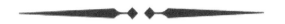

Science Spotlight
Understanding APOE ε4 and
Proactive Dementia Prevention

Knowing if you carry the APOE ε4 variant—the most well-known genetic risk factor for Alzheimer's disease—allows you to take proactive, targeted steps to prevent dementia from becoming a reality. The APOE ε4 variant is linked to increased cholesterol levels and heightened inflammation, which impact both brain and cardiovascular health[1]. With this genetic insight, GeneLean360°'s approach emphasizes specific, science-backed actions to counteract the risks through:

- **Optimized nutrition:** Emphasizing a diet rich in omega-3 fatty acids, antioxidants, and fiber supports brain health, lowers inflammation, and helps maintain optimal cholesterol levels. Foods like fatty fish, nuts, and dark leafy greens are integral in lowering Alzheimer's risk for APOE ε4 carriers.[287]

- **Targeted supplementation:** Key supplements, including omega-3 fatty acids, vitamin D, and CoQ10, support cellular health, reduce brain inflammation, and enhance circulation. For those with APOE ε4, these supplements are powerful tools for protecting brain cells from early degeneration.[288]

- **Structured fitness routine:** Physical activity is one of the most effective ways to support cognitive health by increasing blood flow and reducing inflammation in the brain. Regular cardiovascular and strength training are particularly beneficial for APOE ε4 carriers.[289]

- **Stress-reduction techniques:** Chronic stress is a known trigger for inflammation, which can accelerate cognitive decline. Mindfulness practices, deep breathing, and regular rest help lower stress, supporting a resilient nervous system for those at higher risk.[290]

With these strategic, genetically informed actions, GeneLean360° provides a comprehensive 360-degree defense against not only physical ailments but also mental deterioration, empowering individuals to make impactful lifestyle changes well before symptoms arise.

Phase Three: Personalized Steps for Lisa's Transformation

1. GeneLean360° Tailored Nutrition Plan

For The Vascular Vulnerables™, nutrition plays a pivotal role in reducing cardiovascular strain and supporting long-term wellness. This plan emphasizes foods that support cholesterol management, blood pressure regulation, and vascular health.

What Lisa tried before and why it didn't work:

Low-fat diets or standard low-carb diets: Low-fat or low-carb approaches are popular for weight loss and general health, but they can lack the balance needed for someone with her ACE and APOE genetic profile. These approaches don't directly support cardiovascular flexibility and cholesterol regulation in the targeted way Lisa needs, often leading to only temporary results without significantly impacting her cardiovascular health.

What worked:

High-fiber, low-sodium diet:

- ○ **Fiber-rich whole grains:** Barley and quinoa help manage cholesterol and promote fullness, reducing caloric intake while supporting weight loss.[291]

- ○ **Leafy greens and non-starchy vegetables:** Kale, spinach, broccoli, and Brussels sprouts provide fiber, antioxidants, and potassium, helping regulate blood pressure and protecting against arterial damage.[292]

- ○ **Limit high-sodium foods:** Reducing intake of processed foods, canned soups, and pre-packaged meals helps manage blood pressure, especially critical for individuals with the ACE variant.[293]

Why this works when other approaches did not

For Lisa's genetic profile, specifically addressing her elevated LDL and lipoprotein(a) levels requires a high-fiber approach that also reduces sodium, which helps manage her blood pressure and arterial health. Unlike low-carb or keto diets, the GeneLean360° plan includes foods like barley, flaxseed, and specific leafy greens known to aid cholesterol reduction while targeting the specific genetic pathways affecting her LDL levels.

- **Healthy fats for cholesterol and heart health:**

  - **Omega-3-rich foods:** Salmon, mackerel, chia seeds, flaxseeds, and walnuts reduce inflammation, lower triglycerides, and improve arterial flexibility, benefiting those with APOE ε4 and LPA variants.[294]

  - **Monounsaturated fats:** Olive oil, avocados, and almonds help raise HDL ("good" cholesterol) and support arterial health, improving overall heart resilience.[295]

  - **Limit saturated and trans fats:** Avoiding high-saturated-fat foods like red meat, butter, and processed snacks helps prevent LDL cholesterol buildup in the arteries.[296]

Why this works

For individuals with APOE and LPA variants, these healthy fats promote arterial flexibility, reduce LDL cholesterol, and combat inflammation, essential for long-term heart health. For Lisa, I recommended specific omega-3 and monounsaturated fats based on Lisa's APOE variant, which predisposes her to high LDL cholesterol.

This approach focuses on using omega-3 sources, such as salmon and chia seeds, and monounsaturated fats from olive oil and avocado, both known to improve cholesterol profiles for individuals with APOE variants.

- **Antioxidant-rich foods to reduce inflammation:**

  - **Berries, grapes, and dark chocolate:** These foods are rich in antioxidants that help reduce oxidative stress, a major contributor to arterial plaque formation.[297]

○ **Citrus fruits and red bell peppers:** High in vitamin C, these foods support blood vessel health and boost immune function, which is key to preventing arterial damage.[298]

○ **Green tea and dark leafy greens:** Known for their catechins and flavonoids, green tea and leafy greens improve circulation and protect against arterial plaque buildup.[299]

Why this works

Antioxidants are crucial for individuals like Lisa, reducing inflammation and oxidative damage to arteries, thereby preventing cardiovascular strain and supporting long-term health. Low-carbohydrate diets do not emphasize the importance of anti-inflammatory foods, nor are they tailored to combat the genetic inflammation triggers Lisa faces due to her LPA variant.

For Lisa, I emphasized omega-3-rich foods and antioxidants from sources like fatty fish, walnuts, and berries to lower inflammation and oxidative stress in the vascular system and protect against arterial stiffness and plaque buildup—key for Lisa's cardiovascular health.

2. GeneLean360° Targeted Supplementation™

To support Lisa's cardiovascular resilience, we introduced HeartComplete360°, formulated to address the unique needs of The Vascular Vulnerables™. Lisa's protocol is designed to support blood flow, healthy cholesterol levels, and arterial flexibility—all essential components for cardiovascular strength and endurance.

Key ingredients:

- **Coenzyme Q10 (CoQ10):** CoQ10 is critical for cellular energy and heart muscle function, especially for individuals with elevated cholesterol. It has been shown to improve endothelial function, enhancing vascular health and stamina.[300]

- **Vitamin E:** As a potent antioxidant, vitamin E plays a critical role in protecting cells from oxidative damage, especially in the cardiovascular system. For individuals with elevated lipoprotein(a) and LDL cholesterol levels, vitamin E supports arterial health by preventing cholesterol oxidation, a major contributor to plaque buildup and arterial stiffness.

  o **Why it's essential here:** Given her increased risk for vascular inflammation and oxidative stress, vitamin E reduces the damage from LDL oxidation and inflammation in the arteries, providing crucial protection for long-term cardiovascular health.[301]

Additional supplements:

- **Omega-3 fatty acids:** Known to reduce inflammation, lower triglycerides, and improve arterial flexibility, omega-3s are particularly beneficial for individuals with APOE and LPA variants who need to manage cholesterol and reduce inflammation.[302]

- **Garlic extract:** Garlic has a rich history of use in cardiovascular support, known to reduce blood pressure and improve lipid profiles, making it protective against heart disease.[303]
- **Magnesium:** Magnesium is essential for muscle relaxation, regulating blood pressure, and promoting healthy blood vessel function. It also helps reduce stress, which indirectly benefits cardiovascular health.[304]

3. GeneLean360° Personalized Fitness Plan

A balanced fitness regimen supports cardiovascular health, improves circulation, and builds endurance. For The Vascular Vulnerables™, this approach integrates moderate-intensity cardio, strength training focused on endurance, and flexibility exercises to support vascular health and promote recovery.

- **Moderate-intensity cardio for heart health:**
  - **Frequency:** 4-5 times per week.
  - **Activities:** Brisk walking, cycling, swimming, or rowing.
  - **Duration:** 30-45 minutes per session.

Why: Moderate cardio strengthens the heart, improves circulation, and helps regulate blood pressure. For Lisa, this level of cardio is essential for maintaining cardiovascular resilience.[305]

- **Strength training with focus on endurance:**

  o **Frequency:** 2 times per week.

  o **Focus:** Full-body workouts with lighter weights and higher reps.

  o **Exercises:** Squats, lunges, rows, and planks.

  o **Reps/sets:** 3 sets of 12-15 reps.

Why: Endurance-focused strength training improves circulation and metabolic rate without straining the cardiovascular system. For Lisa, this approach builds stamina, supports heart health, and complements her cardio regimen.[306]

- **Flexibility and mobility work for vascular health:**

  o **Frequency:** 3-4 times per week.

  o **Activities:** Yoga, stretching, or Pilates for 15-20 minutes.

Why: Flexibility exercises improve circulation and reduce vascular stiffness, supporting blood flow. This is essential for Lisa, promoting a balanced fitness routine that aids heart health and resilience.[307]

- **Rest and active recovery emphasis:**

  o **Rest days:** 1-2 days per week, including light activities like walking or gentle stretching.

Why: Recovery days prevent cardiovascular strain, reduce cortisol levels, and support stamina. For Lisa, active rest allows her to recharge without compromising her heart health.[308]

Lisa's Transformation and Breakthrough

After incorporating her personalized GeneLean360° plan, Lisa began to notice empowering changes that transformed her day-to-day life. Her energy levels steadily improved, allowing her to tackle everyday tasks without feeling winded or fatigued. Climbing stairs no longer left her breathless, and she found herself with the stamina to keep up with her kids, something she had dearly missed.

Over four months, Lisa lost *twenty-eight pounds*, achieving sustainable weight loss without feeling deprived or restricted. This weight loss not only improved her physical health, but also gave her a renewed sense of vitality and confidence. As she saw her efforts paying off, her commitment to her health journey grew stronger.

Perhaps most significantly, her blood pressure and cholesterol levels shifted toward optimal ranges, with her blood pressure dropping from 142/90 to 118/75. Her cholesterol levels also improved, signaling enhanced cardiovascular health and a reduced risk of heart disease. These changes reassured Lisa that she was not only losing weight, but also proactively supporting her long-term heart health.

The greatest transformation, however, was in her renewed stamina and confidence. Lisa felt resilient and capable, reassured by the knowledge that she was actively managing her heart health and addressing her genetic predispositions.

"Within three months, my doctor was amazed at the improvements," Lisa shared. "I feel more alive and resilient than I have in years. This journey has been about more than weight loss; it's about reclaiming my health and breaking free from my genetic predispositions."

■ *Lean Genes Blueprint* Entry: Reflecting on Your Cardiovascular Journey

Reflect on your experiences with heart health and weight management.

❖ Have you experienced symptoms like fatigue, high blood pressure, or cholesterol fluctuations?

❖ How do these affect your energy, confidence, and daily life?

❖ Consider how understanding your unique genetic cardiovascular profile could transform your approach to health and wellness.

Chapter 17

The Craving Captives™

Emma's journey demonstrates the powerful link between genetics and uncontrollable food cravings. For The Craving Captives™, weight loss isn't about willpower. It's about understanding how genetic variations in appetite-regulating genes can drive intense urges for high-calorie foods.

Women like Emma often feel trapped in cycles of guilt and shame, battling cravings that seem impossible to control. Through targeted support with the Control360° protocol, Emma broke free from her cravings and transformed her relationship with food. She released thirty-five pounds in five months while reducing her daily cravings from eight to ten episodes to just one or two mild urges. This chapter reveals how you, like Emma, can understand your body's unique appetite signals and finally gain control over cravings that have held you captive.

Have you ever felt powerless against your cravings, no matter how hard you try to resist? Meet Emma, a woman who discovered that understanding her genetic makeup was the key to breaking free from uncontrollable cravings and reclaiming her health. Most importantly, Emma discovered that her struggles weren't a moral failing. They are a genetic predisposition that can be managed.

Phase One: Understanding Emma's Story

Emma, a thirty-nine-year-old marketing executive and mother of three, found herself constantly battling cravings, especially during the late afternoon and evening. Despite her best efforts, she struggled with intense urges for sugary and high-calorie foods.

"It's like there's a switch in my brain that I can't turn off," she confided during our consultation. "I can have a healthy breakfast and lunch, but by 3 p.m., I'm reaching for chocolate or chips. It feels impossible to say no."

For years, Emma had tried various diets, hoping one would curb her cravings. Each attempt left her feeling frustrated and defeated. She felt ashamed of her food choices, and her self-esteem took a hit every time she gave in to a craving. "I feel like I'm failing every day. I can't seem to control myself, no matter how hard I try," she admitted.

What Emma tried before and why it didn't work:

- **Various diets:** Fad diets and restrictive eating plans didn't address the underlying genetic factors driving her cravings.[309]

- **Willpower alone:** Relying solely on willpower led to cycles of guilt and shame when she couldn't resist cravings.[310]

- **Appetite suppressants:** Over-the-counter supplements weren't tailored to her genetic needs and often led to unwanted side effects.[311]

- **Mindful eating practices:** While beneficial, these practices didn't sufficiently counteract the strong biological hunger signals influenced by her genes.[312]

Phase Two: Discovering Emma's Genetic Blueprint

After completing her genetic test as part of joining the GeneLean360° Genetic Gateway, we discovered that Emma fell into a group called The Craving Captives™, with significant variations in her FTO, MC4R, LEPR, and GHRL genes. Understanding her unique genetic predispositions allowed us to design a strategy to help her manage her cravings and take control of her dietary habits.

Emma's genetic test revealed important insights into the underlying causes of her intense cravings and struggles with satiety.

- **FTO (fat mass and obesity-associated gene):** This gene is associated with appetite regulation and preference for high-calorie foods. Individuals with certain FTO variations, like Emma, may experience increased hunger cues and a stronger inclination for calorie-dense foods, making portion control a challenge.[313]

- **MC4R (melanocortin 4 receptor):**MC4R plays a crucial role in controlling energy balance and appetite. Variants in this gene can lead to higher food intake and difficulty feeling full after meals, contributing to persistent cravings.[314]

- **LEPR (leptin receptor gene):** The LEPR gene affects leptin sensitivity, a hormone responsible for signaling fullness. Reduced leptin sensitivity means that the brain doesn't receive strong enough signals to stop eating, which can make individuals feel hungrier, even after consuming sufficient calories.[315]

- **GHRL (ghrelin gene):** Ghrelin, often called the **hunger hormone**, stimulates appetite. Variations in the GHRL gene can increase ghrelin levels, intensifying hunger and craving cues, especially for high-calorie or sugary foods.[316]

Why previous approaches didn't work based on these SNPs:

- **Various diets:** Standard diets didn't address the genetic factors affecting her hunger and satiety signals, leading to persistent cravings despite dietary changes.[317]

- **Willpower alone:** Biological hunger signals influenced by her genetic variations overpowered her willpower, making resistance unsustainable.[318]

- **Appetite suppressants:** Generic suppressants didn't target the specific hormones and pathways affected by her gene variants and sometimes exacerbated her cravings.[319]

- **Mindful eating practices:** While helpful, these practices didn't modify the hormonal imbalances driving her intense hunger and cravings.[320]

I explained to Emma, "Your cravings aren't about lack of discipline—they're deeply connected to your body's unique genetic tendencies. By understanding these signals, we can create a plan that helps you feel more in control."

Relieved and hopeful, Emma saw the first glimmer of a solution tailored to her struggles.

To address Emma's challenges, we went on to explore the key scientific mechanisms behind cravings and satiety:

- **Genetic influence on hunger and satiety:** Genes like FTO and MC4R influence hunger signals and satiety, making individuals with these variants more likely to crave calorie-dense foods. This can result in frequent hunger cues, driving individuals toward snacks that temporarily satisfy but don't provide long-term fullness.[321]

- **Leptin and ghrelin balance:** Leptin, the satiety hormone, and ghrelin play crucial roles in appetite control. For those with LEPR and GHRL variations, this balance is disrupted. Reduced leptin sensitivity prevents the brain from fully recognizing fullness, while elevated ghrelin levels amplify hunger, creating a cycle of intense cravings.[322]

- **Blood sugar regulation:** For The Craving Captives™, blood sugar fluctuations can trigger cravings, especially for high-sugar foods that provide quick energy. These cravings are often short-lived and lead to energy crashes, reinforcing the urge to reach for more calorie-dense foods.[323]

Understanding this science provided Emma with clarity. Her feelings of despair weren't a result of personal failure, but a complex interplay of genetics and biochemistry. Emma's genetic blueprint gave us a clear pathway for managing her cravings through a combination of targeted supplementation, nutrition, and fitness strategies.

Phase Three: Personalized Steps for The Craving Captives™

1. GeneLean360° Tailored Nutrition Plan

What Emma tried before and why it didn't work:

- **Various diets:** Fad diets often involve restrictive eating that doesn't address genetic hunger signals, leading to rebound overeating.[324] [9].
- **Low-calorie diets:** Severe calorie restriction can increase ghrelin levels, intensifying hunger and making cravings worse.[325]

What worked:

The nutrition plan for The Craving Captives™ focuses on balanced meals that stabilize blood sugar, support appetite control, and provide steady energy to reduce cravings.

- **High-protein foods to curb cravings and support satiety:**
  - **Protein with every meal:** Lean proteins such as chicken, turkey, fish, and plant-based proteins like tofu and lentils help stabilize ghrelin, reducing hunger cues and promoting satiety[17].
  - **Protein-packed snacks:** Greek yogurt, cottage cheese, or a handful of nuts help maintain fullness between meals, reducing the likelihood of energy dips that lead to cravings.

Why this works: Protein helps stabilize ghrelin levels, allowing The Craving Captives™ to feel fuller longer, improving their control over appetite and reducing cravings for calorie-dense foods.

- **Fiber-rich foods to prolong fullness and prevent cravings:**
  - **High-fiber vegetables:** Vegetables like broccoli, spinach, and carrots add bulk to meals and provide steady energy release.[326]
  - **Whole grains and legumes:** Complex carbs such as quinoa, barley, and lentils slow digestion and help prevent sugar cravings.

Why this works: Fiber-rich foods help manage blood sugar levels and prolong fullness, essential for The Craving Captives™ to avoid sudden hunger and feel in control throughout the day.[327]

- **Healthy fats to satisfy hunger and balance hormones:**
  - **Omega-3-rich foods:** Fatty fish, walnuts, and flaxseeds support brain health, reduce inflammation, and help manage appetite.[328]
  - **Monosaturated Fats:** Avocado, olive oil, almonds provide sustained energy and enhances satiety.

Why this works: Healthy fats offer a lasting energy source and hormone balance, keeping The Craving Captives™ satisfied and less reliant on high-calorie snacks.

- **Low-glycemic carbohydrates to avoid blood sugar spikes:**

  o **Low-glycemic carbs:** Foods like lentils and berries release energy slowly, preventing sudden spikes and crashes that intensify cravings.[329]

  o **Limit sugary and refined carbs:** High-sugar snacks and processed foods lead to rapid energy spikes, followed by crashes, which intensify cravings.

Why: Low-glycemic carbs keep blood sugar stable, reducing cravings for quick, calorie-dense fixes.

2. GeneLean360° Targeted Supplementation™

What Emma tried before and why it didn't work:

- **Generic appetite suppressants:** Over-the-counter options rarely address the genetic nuances that drive intense cravings, often leading to minimal results or unwanted side effects.[330]

- **Untargeted supplements:** Without focusing on the genes influencing hunger and satiety, supplements can miss the mark, failing to stabilize the hormones and neurotransmitters involved in cravings and fullness.[331]

To support Emma in managing her cravings and achieving satiety, we introduced the Control360° Tea, a precise blend of botanicals selected for their genetic-aligned benefits. Unlike generic products, Control360° Tea considers variations in FTO, MC4R, LEPR, and GHRL, working in harmony with your body's unique blueprint. By promoting balanced blood sugar, supporting leptin sensitivity, and calming stress-induced hunger, this tea helps reduce the intensity and frequency of cravings.

Key Ingredients in Control360° Tea:

- **Rooibos (Aspalathus linearis)**

Known for its natural sweetness and antioxidant properties, Rooibos supports healthy leptin signaling and reduces oxidative stress that can aggravate hunger cues.[332]

Why it works: Rooibos helps balance leptin sensitivity, improving your body's ability to recognize fullness and curbing the drive to overeat, particularly important for individuals with LEPR variations.

- **Calendula Petals (Calendula officinalis)**

Calendula's anti-inflammatory properties enhance gut health and hormone signaling.[333] Improved gut health is linked to more stable ghrelin levels, reducing persistent hunger pangs.

Why it works: By fostering a healthier internal environment, Calendula supports balanced hunger hormones, aiding those with GHRL variations who struggle with unrelenting appetite surges.

- **Cinnamon (Cinnamomum verum)**

Cinnamon helps regulate blood sugar by improving insulin sensitivity, stabilizing energy and preventing the rapid spikes and crashes that trigger cravings.[334]

Why it works: For FTO and MC4R variants that predispose you to prefer high-calorie foods, stable blood sugar reduces the pull toward sugary snacks, making it easier to resist temptation.

- **Licorice Root (Glycyrrhiza glabra)**

Naturally sweet without adding sugar, licorice root can help modulate cortisol levels, reducing stress-induced cravings.[335] Lower stress equals fewer emotional eating episodes.

Why it works: Individuals who turn to high-calorie treats under stress benefit from licorice root's ability to smooth out emotional triggers, aligning with LEPR-driven hunger signals.

- **Chicory Root (Cichorium intybus)**

Rich in inulin, a prebiotic fiber, chicory root supports gut flora balance. A healthier gut environment can improve nutrient absorption and fullness cues.[336]

Why it works: By enhancing feelings of satiety, chicory root helps counter the persistent hunger seen in GHRL and LEPR variants, making it easier to maintain dietary control.

Why this approach works:

Control360° Tea tackles the root biochemical and genetic factors driving The Craving Captives™. While Emma's previous attempts failed due to generic methods, this tea uses scientifically supported ingredients chosen for their ability to influence leptin and ghrelin balance, improve insulin sensitivity, and enhance gut health. This synergy stabilizes hunger signals, reduces emotional cravings, and makes it easier to maintain consistent, healthier eating habits.

For Emma, Control360° Tea offered a daily ritual that didn't feel like deprivation. Instead, it tasted soothing and naturally satisfying, reinforcing her body's hormonal and metabolic balance. Over time, she noticed fewer afternoon sugar cravings, improved portion control, and a sense of empowerment that came from understanding—and mastering—her genetic blueprint.

3. GeneLean360° Personalized Fitness Plan

What Emma tried before and why it didn't work:

- **Inconsistent exercise routines:** Lack of a structured plan led to minimal impact on insulin sensitivity and stress levels, which are crucial for appetite control.[337]

- **High-intensity workouts:** Overly intense exercises increased cortisol levels, potentially exacerbating hunger and cravings.[338] She left her workouts starving! Her intense cravings didn't stand a chance.

What worked instead:

A structured fitness routine supports appetite control by improving insulin sensitivity, managing stress, and stabilizing energy. The following plan is tailored to help The Craving Captives™ balance their hunger and reduce emotional eating triggers.

- **Moderate-intensity cardio for fat burn and craving reduction:**
  - ○ **Frequency:** 3-4 days per week.
  - ○ **Activities:** Brisk walking, cycling, swimming, or low-impact dance.

○ **Duration:** 30-45 minutes per session.

Why: Moderate cardio helps release endorphins, improving mood and reducing cravings for comfort foods. Improved insulin sensitivity also helps The Craving Captives™ control blood sugar.[339]

- **Strength training to boost metabolism and stabilize blood sugar:**

○ **Frequency:** 2-3 days per week.

○ **Focus:** Full-body workouts with exercises like squats, lunges, push-ups, and rows.

○ **Reps/sets:** 3 sets of 10-12 reps with moderate weights.

Why: Building lean muscle increases metabolic rate and improves blood sugar control, essential for reducing the frequency and intensity of cravings.[340]

- **Mindfulness practices to curb emotional eating:**

○ **Frequency:** 2-3 times per week.

○ **Activities:** Yoga, meditation, or mindful breathing for 15-20 minutes.

Why: Mindfulness helps reduce stress and improve emotional regulation, allowing The Craving Captives™ to manage cravings with greater control. Lower stress levels also reduce cortisol, which is linked to increased hunger.[341]

- **Hydration to control hunger and support satiety:**

○ **Hydration goal:** 80 ounces of water daily, with 20 ounces before each meal.

Why: Staying hydrated reduces mistaken hunger cues caused by thirst. Drinking water before meals promotes fullness and reduces the tendency to overeat.[342]

Emma's Breakthrough: From Cravings to Control

Emma's transformation was nothing short of life-changing. Through a combination of Control360° Tea and a personalized nutrition and fitness plan, she took back control of her cravings—and her life.

At the start of her journey, Emma was battling eight to ten intense cravings for sugary snacks every day. But over time, those cravings dwindled to just one or two mild urges.

"It feels so freeing," she shared, reflecting on how it felt to no longer be ruled by constant hunger. With her blood sugar finally balanced and a steady energy flow throughout the day, she no longer experienced the exhausting energy crashes that once drained her.

Over five months, Emma lost *thirty-five pounds*—and she did it without feeling deprived. But perhaps the most powerful change wasn't the number on the scale. It was her new relationship with food. She no longer felt like hunger had control over her. Instead, she could enjoy meals with peace and balance.

"Realizing my cravings were connected to my genetics changed everything," Emma explained. "For the first time, I feel in control, and it's empowering to know I can manage this."

I created Control360° Tea because I know firsthand how exhausting it is to feel controlled by cravings. No matter how much willpower you summon, cravings can feel relentless—and that's because they're often rooted in your genetics. This tea is designed to work with your body's unique needs, helping you reclaim control without constant struggle.

If you're ready to experience freedom from cravings, visit genelean360.com/store and take the first step toward lasting change.

▣ *Lean Genes Blueprint* Entry: Reflecting on Your Craving Patterns

❖ Do you often experience intense cravings or frequent hunger cues?

❖ What times of day or specific situations tend to trigger these feelings?

❖ How could understanding your unique genetic appetite signals change your approach to health and weight management?

Chapter 18

The Gut Imbalanced™

For The Gut Imbalanced™, weight loss isn't just about calories. It's about healing from the inside out. Olivia's journey reflects the frustrating reality many women face when their gut works against them. Every meal became a source of anxiety, leaving her bloated, uncomfortable, and trapped in a cycle of digestive distress. Like many of The Gut Imbalanced™, she felt betrayed by her body, watching as stomach issues sabotaged her weight loss efforts despite her dedication to healthy eating.

Olivia's story transformed when she discovered the genetic roots of her digestive struggles. By aligning with her body's unique needs and healing her gut through targeted strategies, she achieved what once seemed impossible—losing fifty-six pounds and fifteen inches in six months. More importantly, she found freedom from the digestive issues that had controlled her life. This chapter reveals how you too can unlock your body's ability to heal, digest, and thrive by understanding The Gut Imbalanced™ genetic blueprint for yourself.

Have you ever felt your digestion is sabotaging you, no matter how healthy you eat or how diligently you exercise? Meet Olivia, a woman who discovered that understanding her genetic makeup as one of The Gut Imbalanced™ was the key to unlocking her body's potential and achieving lasting change.

Phase One: Understanding Olivia's Story

Olivia stared at her reflection in the mirror, her hands resting gently on her bloated stomach. It was the same discomfort she felt after nearly every meal—an uncomfortable fullness that seemed to sap her energy and spirit. At thirty-eight, she was tired of feeling this way. Despite her best efforts to eat healthily and stay active, her digestion seemed to betray her at every turn.

When she pushed her plate away at dinner, half-eaten, her son asked, "Mommy, aren't you hungry?"

"I am, sweetie," she replied with a forced smile. "My stomach just doesn't feel good."

Meals had become a source of anxiety. The unpredictability of her digestion left her cautious about what she ate, yet nothing seemed to make a difference. Bloating, irregularity, and a constant feeling of heaviness were her daily companions. Exercise, once a stress reliever, now felt like a chore as her energy levels plummeted.

"I feel heavy and tired all the time," Olivia confided during our initial consultation. "It's like nothing digests properly. I don't understand what's wrong with me."

Her weight loss journey was equally frustrating. Despite eating "all the right things," the scale wouldn't budge. The digestive discomfort affected her motivation to exercise, and she often craved comfort foods to soothe her upset stomach—only to feel worse afterward.

The cycle seemed endless, and Olivia was losing hope. "I just want to feel normal," she said softly. "Is that too much to ask?"

Scrolling through social media one night, she stumbled upon a testimonial from someone who had overcome similar issues through a program called GeneLean360°. Intrigued by the mention of genetic insights into gut health, Olivia decided to reach out.

Phase Two: Discovering Olivia's Genetic Blueprint

At her consultation, I recall distinctly just how exasperated Olivia was.

"I've tried everything—gluten-free, dairy-free, low-FODMAP diets," she explained. "Nothing gives me lasting relief. I'm constantly bloated, and it's affecting every aspect of my life."

"Olivia, your symptoms are real," I said to validate her experience. "And they have a root cause. Let's explore what's happening at a deeper level."

We decided to conduct genetic testing to uncover any underlying factors contributing to her digestive issues and weight loss resistance. The results were revealing. Olivia belonged to a group I call The Gut Imbalanced™, characterized by specific genetic variations affecting gut health:

- **FUT2 (fucosyltransferase 2):**

    o **Role:** Influences the composition of gut microbiota by affecting the secretion of certain sugars that beneficial bacteria feed on.[343]

o **Olivia's variant:** Reduced activity of FUT2, leading to lower levels of beneficial bacteria like *Bifidobacteria*.

o **Impact:** A less diverse microbiome can impair digestion, nutrient absorption, and immune function.[344]

- **MCM6 (minichromosome maintenance complex component 6):**

o **Role:** Regulates the expression of the lactase enzyme responsible for digesting lactose in dairy products.[345]

o **Olivia's variant:** Lactase non-persistence (lactose intolerance), resulting in difficulty digesting lactose.

o **Impact:** Consuming dairy led to bloating, gas, and discomfort due to undigested lactose fermenting in the gut.[346]

- **IL10 (interleukin 10):**

o **Role:** Encodes an anti-inflammatory cytokine that regulates immune responses in the gut.[347]

o **Olivia's variant:** Lower expression of IL10, leading to increased gut inflammation.

o **Impact:** Heightened inflammatory responses can damage the gut lining, affecting digestion and promoting discomfort.[348]

Why previous approaches didn't work based on these SNPs:

- **Gluten-free and dairy-free diets:** While eliminating gluten and dairy can help some, Olivia's issues were rooted in her microbiome diversity and inflammation, not just food sensitivities.[349]

- **Low-FODMAP diets:** Restricting FODMAPs reduced some symptoms temporarily but didn't address her underlying bacterial imbalances and inflammation.[350]

- **Over-the-counter probiotics:** Generic probiotics lacked the specific strains needed to address her unique microbiome deficiencies caused by the FUT2 variant.[351]

With this genetic insight, Olivia could finally understand why her gut had been a constant source of discomfort. "I'm not just imagining it," she said. "There's an actual reason for these issues."

"Exactly," I affirmed. "Your body has been sending signals that we can now interpret. Understanding your genetic blueprint allows us to create a plan tailored just for you."

To fully grasp Olivia's struggle, let's delve into the science behind how gut health impacts weight management and overall well-being:

- **Microbiome diversity:** A balanced microbiome is crucial for nutrient absorption and immune function. Variations in FUT2 gene can reduce beneficial bacteria like *Bifidobacteria*, can reduce beneficial bacteria diversity, making it harder to support metabolism and immune health. Targeted probiotics and prebiotics can restore gut balance and improve digestive function for The Gut Imbalanced™.

- **Lactose tolerance and digestion:** MCM6 impacts the production of lactase, the enzyme that digests lactose. For those with variations in this gene, undigested lactose can ferment in the gut, causing bloating and discomfort. Identifying and reducing lactose can alleviate these symptoms and promote gut comfort.

- **Inflammation and gut health:** Inflammation can damage the gut lining, leading to nutrient malabsorption and digestive discomfort. IL10 plays a role in regulating inflammation, and anti-inflammatory strategies, including diet and supplements, can be beneficial for those with IL10 variations.

By focusing on gut balance, Olivia could work with her body instead of against it, finally seeing a clear path to lasting wellness.

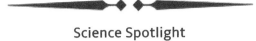

Science Spotlight
Understanding your Microbiome

The term *microbiome* might sound scientific, but it simply refers to the vast community of tiny organisms—bacteria, fungi, and other microbes—that live in and on our bodies, especially in our digestive system. Think of your gut microbiome as a bustling city filled with trillions of microorganisms, each playing a role in keeping you healthy.

These microbes aren't just passive passengers; they actively help you digest food, absorb nutrients, and protect against harmful bacteria. They even communicate with your immune system and produce vitamins essential for health. A healthy, balanced microbiome can help you maintain energy, boost mood, and support metabolism.

How does it affect weight loss and digestion?

Your microbiome plays a crucial role in weight management and digestive health. Studies show that a diverse and balanced microbiome supports better digestion, aids in nutrient absorption, and can even help regulate appetite. Conversely, an imbalanced microbiome (often due to stress, diet, or genetic factors) may contribute to digestive discomfort, cravings, and stubborn weight gain.

Every person's microbiome is unique, shaped by factors like genetics and lifestyle. By learning about your specific gut bacteria needs, you can make personalized dietary and lifestyle choices that foster a healthier microbiome, aligning your body with your wellness goals.

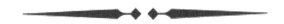

Phase Three: Personalized Steps for The Gut Imbalanced™

1. GeneLean360° Tailored Nutrition Plan

What Olivia tried before and why it didn't work:

Gluten-free and dairy-free diets: These diets didn't address her specific bacterial imbalances and inflammation. Eliminating gluten and dairy alone wasn't enough.[352]

Low-FODMAP diet: While it reduced some symptoms, it was too restrictive and didn't promote the growth of beneficial bacteria needed for long-term gut health.[353]

What worked:

Emphasizing foods that support gut health, restore microbial balance, and reduce inflammation to enhance nutrient absorption and digestive wellness.

High-fiber, prebiotic-rich diet:

○ **Prebiotic foods:** Asparagus, garlic, onions, leeks, and bananas provide fuel for beneficial gut bacteria, supporting microbiome health.[354]

○ **High-fiber vegetables and whole grains:** Foods like artichokes, broccoli, Brussels sprouts and barley aid in digestion and promote regularity.

○ **Limit high-FODMAP foods if sensitive:** Certain high-FODMAP foods can cause discomfort; reducing them may improve gut comfort.

Why this works: Prebiotics nourish beneficial bacteria like *Bifidobacteria*, and fiber promotes regularity, essential for The Gut Imbalanced™ needing balanced gut health to enhance nutrient absorption.

Probiotic foods to introduce beneficial bacteria:

○ **Fermented foods:** Yogurt, kefir (non-dairy options if lactose intolerant), sauerkraut, kimchi, and miso introduce probiotics that foster a balanced microbiome.[355]

○ **Start with small portions:** Introduce these foods gradually to prevent digestive upset for sensitive individuals.

Why this works: Probiotic foods support a healthy microbiome and improve digestion, enhancing the immune response and nutrient absorption for The Gut Imbalanced™.

Anti-inflammatory foods to soothe the gut:

○ **Omega-3-rich foods:** Include salmon, chia seeds, flaxseeds, and walnuts to reduce gut inflammation associated with IL10 variations.[356]

○ **Ginger and turmeric:** Add to meals or teas for digestive support and anti-inflammatory benefits.

○ **Limit processed foods and sugars:** Avoid added sugars and artificial sweeteners, which can disrupt the microbiome.

Why this works: Anti-inflammatory foods reduce gut inflammation, supporting the gut lining and digestive health, essential for The Gut Imbalanced™.

Lactose-free alternatives:

o **Inclusion:** Almond milk, coconut yogurt.

o **Why:** Avoid lactose to prevent discomfort from MCM6-related lactose intolerance.[357]

2. GeneLean360° Targeted Supplementation™

What Olivia tried before and why it didn't work:

Generic probiotics: Lacked specific strains needed to address her FUT2 variant and didn't survive stomach acid to reach the gut effectively.[358]

Over-the-counter digestive enzymes: Provided temporary relief but didn't address underlying microbiome imbalances or inflammation.[359]

What worked:

To support Olivia's gut health, we introduced Gutbalance360°, a probiotic supplement designed to restore gut balance and improve digestive function. This blend targets the specific challenges of The Gut Imbalanced™, providing a range of beneficial bacterial strains to address microbiome imbalances and support nutrient absorption.

Key ingredients:

▪ **Lactobacillus acidophilus (La-14):** Supports healthy digestion and boosts the immune system by fostering a balanced gut environment.[360]

- **Lactobacillus paracasei (Lpc-37):** Known for its role in promoting gut health and supporting digestion, particularly in individuals with microbiome imbalances.[361]

- **Bifidobacterium bifidum (Bb-02):** Aids in breaking down complex carbs and helps reduce digestive discomfort, supporting efficient digestion.[362]

- **Bifidobacterium lactis (BI-04):** Supports immune health and improves lactose digestion, making it ideal for those with MCM6 variations.[363]

- **Lactobacillus plantarum (Lp-115):** Known for its anti-inflammatory properties and ability to support the gut lining, helping with IL10-related inflammation.[364]

- **Lactobacillus rhamnosus (GG):** Enhances gut barrier integrity, improves digestion, and supports immune response.[365]

Why this approach works:

Gutbalance360° provides targeted probiotic strains that specifically address The Gut Imbalanced™ genetic variations, fostering a balanced microbiome, improving digestion, and reducing inflammation—something generic supplements failed to achieve.

3. GeneLean360° Personalized Fitness Plan

What Olivia tried before and why it didn't work:

- **High-intensity workouts:** Increased cortisol levels, exacerbating inflammation and digestive issues.[366]

- **Inconsistent exercise due to discomfort:** Lack of regular activity hindered digestion and stress management.

What worked instead:

This gentle fitness plan supports digestion, gut health, and stress reduction.

- **Low to moderate-intensity cardio:**
    - **Frequency:** 3-4 times per week.
    - **Activities:** Walking, cycling, or swimming at a moderate pace.
    - **Duration:** 30-45 minutes per session.

Why it works: Low to moderate cardio supports gut motility and reduces inflammation, without causing stress that can disrupt digestion.[367]

- **Core strengthening and postural exercises:**
    - **Frequency:** 2 times per week.
    - **Focus:** Exercises like planks, bird-dogs, and leg raises, emphasizing controlled breathing.
    - **Reps/sets:** 2-3 sets of 10-12 reps with attention to form.

Why it works: A strong core supports digestive health by improving posture and relieving pressure on digestive organs.[368]

- **Mind-body exercises to support gut-brain connection:**
  - ○ **Frequency:** 3 times per week.
  - ○ **Activities:** Yoga, tai chi, or Pilates for 15-30 minutes.

Why it works: Mind-body practices support the gut-brain connection and reduce stress, which can significantly impact gut health and alleviates digestive discomfort.[369]

4. Lifestyle Modifications

- **Stress management:**
  - ○ **Techniques:** Deep-breathing exercises, mindfulness meditation.
  - ○ **Why:** Chronic stress exacerbates gut inflammation and discomfort.[370]

- **Sleep hygiene:**
  - ○ **Goal:** 7-8 hours of quality sleep per night.
  - ○ **Why:** Sleep supports gut health and overall recovery.[371]

- **Hydration:**
  - ○ **Goal:** At least 80 ounces of water daily.
  - ○ **Why:** Adequate hydration aids digestion and nutrient absorption.[372]

Implementation plan:

- **Daily routine:**

    o   Incorporate stress-reduction techniques before meals and bedtime.

    o   Establish a consistent sleep schedule.

    o   Sip water throughout the day.

Why this approach works:

Lifestyle factors like stress and sleep have profound impacts on gut health. By addressing these areas, Olivia supports her body's natural healing processes.

Olivia's Transformation and Breakthrough

The changes didn't happen overnight, but within weeks, Olivia began to notice significant improvements. Her bloating diminished, and meals no longer filled her with dread.

"I had dinner last night and felt... normal," she shared excitedly during a follow-up. "No discomfort, no bloating. I can't remember the last time that happened."

As months passed, the scale started to reflect her efforts—a loss of *fifty-six pounds* in six months. But more importantly, Olivia felt revitalized. Her energy levels soared, and she reconnected with activities she loved.

"I have the energy to play with my son again," she beamed. "I feel like myself for the first time in years."

Her journey was a testament to the power of personalized health strategies. By understanding her genetic blueprint, Olivia moved from frustration to empowerment, reclaiming not just her health but her joy in life.

Her story resonates with many women silently battling similar struggles—feeling trapped by digestive issues and weight that won't shift despite their best efforts. If you relate to her journey, remember that you're not alone, and there's a path forward tailored just for you.

Exploring your genetic blueprint can unveil the root causes of your digestive struggles. By aligning your health strategies with your body's unique needs, you can heal from the inside out and step into a life of vitality and comfort.

■ *Lean Genes Blueprint* **Entry: Reflecting on Your Gut Health Journey**

Reflect on your experiences with digestive issues:

- ❖ Have you faced bloating, irregularity, or fatigue?
- ❖ How have these symptoms impacted your daily life and weight loss efforts?
- ❖ Consider how understanding your unique genetic gut profile could change your approach.

I created Gutbalance360° after recognizing a significant pattern in the women I worked with. Many had variations in their FUT2, MCM6, and IL10 genes, impacting their gut health and experiencing persistent symptoms like bloating, fatigue, and weight gain.

For these women, traditional methods weren't enough. With Gutbalance360°, we've seen women achieve remarkable improvements in digestion, energy levels, and weight management.

To discover how this system can support your unique gut health needs, visit genelean360.com/store today.

Chapter 19

The Carb Converters™

For The Carb Converters™, the path to lasting weight loss isn't about saying goodbye to pasta nights or giving up pizza with friends. It's about discovering the freedom to enjoy carbs in harmony with their unique genetic makeup. Felicia's story resonates with countless women who've been told that carbs are the enemy, only to find themselves trapped in cycles of restriction and intense cravings. Like many of The Carb Converters™, she felt forced to choose between enjoying life's pleasures and achieving her health goals.

Everything changed when she discovered her genetic blueprint revealed an unexpected truth: her body was designed to process carbohydrates efficiently. By working with her natural genetic strengths instead of fighting them, Felicia achieved what seemed impossible—losing forty-eight pounds in just five months while still enjoying her weekly pizza nights and occasional glass of wine. Her transformation wasn't just about the numbers; it was about finding freedom in her relationship with food.

This chapter reveals how you too can unlock your body's natural ability to thrive while still enjoying the foods you love, proving that sustainable weight loss doesn't have to mean saying goodbye to life's simple pleasures.

Have you ever felt trapped between your love for carbs and your desire to lose weight, constantly battling cravings and feelings of deprivation? Meet Felicia, a woman who discovered that understanding her genetic makeup as one of The Carb Converters™ was the key to achieving lasting weight loss without giving up the foods she loves.

Phase One: Understanding Felicia's Story

Felicia loved food—especially carbs. A slice of pizza shared with friends, a creamy bowl of pasta on a cold night, a glass of wine that signaled the end of a long week—these were her simple pleasures. But everywhere she turned, the message was clear: "Carbs are the enemy if you want to lose weight."

Desperate to make a change, she tried cutting out carbs completely. The result? She felt deprived, her cravings intensified, and her mood plummeted. She'd often lie in bed, unable to shake the gnawing feeling that she was punishing herself for simply wanting to enjoy her life.

As Felicia brushed her teeth, she noticed her engagement ring lying on the counter, a habit she'd fallen into to avoid the uncomfortable squeeze on her swollen fingers. She tried to ignore the reflection in the mirror— lately, she barely recognized herself. The woman staring back seemed tired, worn down, and heavier in ways that felt both literal and metaphorical.

As she picked out clothes each morning, the frustration mounted. Her favorite jeans now pinched her waist so tightly by midday, they left marks on her skin, and her go-to tops stretched across her back and stomach in a way that made her feel self-conscious. Loose clothing became her daily armor, a way to hide the parts of herself she felt uncomfortable with.

Felicia's confidence had begun to impact other areas of her life. She'd skip social events with friends, making excuses about being too busy, when, really, she dreaded the embarrassment of feeling like the "bigger friend."

She remembered a recent flash of panic when she'd had to ask for a seatbelt extender on a flight. It was the first time, and the memory lingered, haunting her. With an upcoming trip, she found herself silently praying that she wouldn't need one again—or worse, that she wouldn't need to buy the seat next to her just to feel comfortable.

Even at work, she felt her discomfort creeping in. In meetings, she would sit strategically to avoid anyone noticing how her blouse stretched when she moved. She no longer felt like the confident, vibrant woman she used to be. And it wasn't just physical—she felt weighed down in spirit.

Phase Two: Discovering Felicia's Genetic Blueprint

At our consultation, I recall Felicia bravely and openly voicing her frustrations. "I just want to enjoy my life and still be healthy," she said, her voice barely hiding the mix of hope and frustration. "Is it too much to ask to have pizza and wine and still lose weight?"

Her words hung in the air, and she looked down, clearly embarrassed by her own longing.

For Felicia, this wasn't just about weight. It was about reclaiming her sense of self. She was tired of feeling trapped between her love for food and her desire to be healthy. That battle was taking its toll.

"I've tried every low-carb diet out there," she sighed. "Keto, Atkins, you name it. I lose a few pounds, but I can't stick with it. I end up feeling miserable and bingeing on carbs even more."

I smiled reassuringly. "Felicia, what if I told you that your body might actually thrive on carbohydrates?"

Her eyes widened. "Is that even possible?"

"We can find out," I replied. "Let's look at your genetic blueprint to see how your body processes carbs."

We decided to conduct genetic testing to uncover any underlying factors influencing her metabolism and relationship with carbohydrates.

The results were enlightening. Felicia belonged to a group I call The Carb Converters™, characterized by specific genetic variations that enable efficient carbohydrate metabolism:

- **PPARG (peroxisome proliferator-activated receptor gamma):** This gene is essential in how our bodies store and use energy. Specifically, PPARG influences the development of fat cells, known as adipocyte differentiation,[373] by helping immature cells become fully developed fat cells that can store energy. It also plays a key role in glucose metabolism, the process by which our bodies use sugar for energy.

  People with certain PPARG variants have improved insulin sensitivity—meaning their bodies respond better to insulin, allowing them to use carbohydrates efficiently as energy instead of storing them as fat.[374]

- **ADRB2 (beta-2 adrenergic receptor):** This gene plays a role in how our bodies break down fat (a process called lipolysis) and generate heat or energy (known as thermogenesis) in response to food and activity.[375] These processes are essential for burning calories and managing weight. Certain variations in the ADRB2 gene can impact an individual's metabolic rate and how effectively their body burns fat for energy. Felicia's specific ADRB2 variant indicated that her body is well-equipped to handle carbohydrates, especially when she balances them with proteins and healthy fats.[376]

- **FABP2 (fatty acid-binding protein 2):** FABP2 is involved in the intestinal absorption of fatty acids.[377] Certain FABP2 variants increase the absorption rate of fatty acids, affecting how the body handles dietary fats and carbs. Felicia's variant indicates a balanced absorption, allowing for moderate carb and fat intake without negative effects on weight.[378]

- **SLC2A2 (glucose transporter type 2):** Also known as GLUT2, this gene encodes a glucose transporter responsible for glucose uptake in the liver and pancreas.[379] Variations can impact glucose sensing and insulin secretion.[380] Felicia's variant allows for efficient glucose uptake and utilization, supporting stable energy levels.

Why previous approaches didn't work based on these SNPs:

- **Strict low-carb diets (e.g., keto, Atkins):** These diets deprived Felicia of carbs her body was genetically primed to use efficiently, leading to low energy and intense cravings.[381] Restricting carbs disrupted her metabolism, causing her body to store fat instead of burning it effectively.

- **Calorie restriction:** Severely limiting calories slowed her metabolic rate, counteracting the benefits of her ADRB2 variant.[382] Her body became more efficient at conserving energy, making weight loss harder.

- **High-fat diets:** Excessive fat intake didn't align with her FABP2 variant, potentially leading to fat accumulation.[383] Her body couldn't process the high fat load efficiently, undermining weight loss efforts.

Felicia looked at the results with a mix of disbelief and excitement. "So, you're saying I can eat carbs and still lose weight?"

"Exactly," I affirmed. "Your body is designed to process carbohydrates efficiently. By working with your genetic strengths, we can create a plan that allows you to enjoy the foods you love while achieving your health goals."

Understanding these genetic factors provided clarity for Felicia. Her body was designed to handle carbohydrates efficiently, especially when consumed mindfully and paired with supportive nutrients.

To appreciate how Felicia's genetics enable her to enjoy carbs without negative consequences, it's essential to delve into the mechanisms at play:

- **Insulin sensitivity and glucose uptake:** PPARG and SLC2A2 variants can enhance insulin sensitivity and glucose uptake into cells, promoting the use of glucose for immediate energy rather than storing it as fat.

- **Fat oxidation and energy expenditure:** ADRB2 influences how the body oxidizes fats and carbs for energy. Efficient ADRB2 function supports a higher metabolic rate and increased thermogenesis, aiding in weight management even with carb intake.[384]

- **Nutrient absorption and utilization:** FABP2 affects the absorption of fatty acids, balancing the intake of fats and carbs. This balance is crucial for optimal energy utilization and preventing excess fat accumulation.[385]

By aligning her diet and lifestyle with these genetic strengths, Felicia could enjoy her favorite carb-rich foods while supporting her weight management goals.

Part Three: Personalized Steps for Felicia's Transformation

1. GeneLean360° Tailored Nutrition Plan

What Felicia tried before and why it didn't work:

Strict low-carb diets (keto, Atkins): Deprived her of carbs her body was designed to use efficiently, leading to low energy, cravings, and unsustainable eating patterns.[386]

High-fat diets: Excessive fat intake didn't align with her FABP2 variant, potentially causing fat storage instead of fat burning.[387]

What worked:

Embracing quality carbohydrates:

- ○ **Whole grains:** Incorporate quinoa, barley, and bulgur These complex carbs provide sustained energy and are rich in fiber, which slows glucose absorption·

- ○ **Fruits and vegetables:** Focus on a variety of colorful fruits and veggies, especially those with a low glycemic index, such as berries, apples, and leafy greens.

Why this works: High-quality carbs provide essential nutrients and fiber, supporting stable blood sugar levels and efficient metabolism.

Balance macronutrients:

- ○ **Lean proteins:** Include chicken, turkey, fish, legumes, and tofu to promote satiety and muscle maintenance.

- ○ **Healthy fats:** Add sources like avocados, nuts, seeds, and olive oil to meals to enhance nutrient absorption and provide essential fatty acids.

Why this works: Balancing carbs with protein and healthy fats slows digestion, promotes fullness, and stabilizes blood sugar, aligning with Felicia's genetic profile.

Mindful indulgences:

- o **Moderation, not deprivation:** No one loses weight eating boxes of pizza every day. (This is binge eating, which can happen when we are overly restrictive). However, The Carb Converters™ can enjoy pizza and wine by balancing them with nutrient-dense choices.

- o **Portion awareness:** Practice mindful eating, paying attention to hunger and fullness cues to prevent overeating.

Why this works: Satisfying cravings in moderation prevents feelings of deprivation, reduces the likelihood of bingeing, and supports sustainable eating habits.

Blood sugar support:

- o **Include fiber-rich foods:** Aim for a high intake of dietary fiber to slow glucose absorption and promote gut health.

- o **Use the Release Tea:** Incorporate the Release Tea to support blood sugar regulation and reduce post-meal glucose spikes.

Why this works: Maintaining stable blood sugar levels prevents energy crashes and excessive insulin release, supporting weight management.

2. GeneLean360° Targeted Supplementation™

To further support Felicia's carbohydrate metabolism and overall wellness, we introduced the GeneLean360° Release Tea, a carefully crafted herbal blend designed to enhance metabolic function, support digestion, and balance energy levels.

Key ingredients:

- **Rooibos tea:** Rich in antioxidants like aspalathin, rooibos tea has been shown to improve blood glucose levels and reduce oxidative stress. It supports digestion and reduces inflammation, aiding those with genetic variations affecting fat storage.

- **Dandelion root:** Contains inulin, a prebiotic fiber that supports gut health and may improve insulin sensitivity. It aids detoxification and helps curb cravings, beneficial for those with insulin resistance tendencies.

- **Gymnema sylvestre leaf:** Known as the **sugar destroyer**, it can reduce sugar absorption in the intestines and may help regenerate insulin-producing cells. It addresses cravings linked to increased appetite genes.

- **Cinnamon bark:** A natural metabolism booster! The cinnamaldehyde in it helps your body use carbs better and makes it easier for cells to take in glucose. This reduces insulin resistance, helping keep blood sugar levels balanced.

- **Gynostemma pentaphyllum leaf:** An adaptogenic herb that may help regulate metabolism and support energy balance. It enhances metabolic rate complementing ADRB2 variants.

Why this approach works: The Release Tea provides natural, targeted support for Felicia's genetic strengths, enhancing her body's ability to metabolize carbohydrates and maintain energy levels without interfering with her natural processes.

3. GeneLean360° Personalized Fitness Plan

What Felicia tried before and why it didn't work:

- **HIIT:** Led to burnout and increased appetite, causing her to overeat.

- **Excessive cardio:** Prolonged sessions increased cortisol levels, potentially promoting fat storage.

Felicia's fitness plan complemented her nutrition strategy, focusing on activities that enhance carbohydrate utilization and overall metabolic health.

- **Moderate-intensity cardiovascular exercise:**
  - **Frequency:** 4-5 times per week.
  - **Activities:** Brisk walking, cycling, swimming, or dance classes.
  - **Duration:** 30-60 minutes per session.

Why this works: Regular cardio improves insulin sensitivity, increases glucose uptake by muscles, and enhances cardiovascular health.

- **Resistance training:**
  - **Frequency:** 2-3 times per week.
  - **Exercises:** Full-body workouts targeting major muscle groups with exercises like squats, lunges, push-ups, and rows.
  - **Reps/sets:** 2-3 sets of 8-12 reps.

Why this works: Building lean muscle mass increases resting metabolic rate and improves glucose metabolism, essential for effective carb utilization.

- **Flexibility and mind-body practices:**
  - **Frequency:** 1-2 times per week.
  - **Activities:** Yoga, Pilates, or stretching routines.

Why this works: These practices enhance flexibility, reduce stress, and support hormonal balance, which can influence appetite and metabolism.

- **Active lifestyle:**
  - **Incorporate movement:** Take the stairs, walk during breaks, and engage in recreational activities.

Why: Increasing daily movement boosts overall energy expenditure and promotes metabolic health.

Felicia's Transformation and Breakthrough

With her personalized nutrition and fitness plan, supported by the Release Tea, Felicia began to see significant changes. She enjoyed her favorite meals without guilt, experienced steady energy throughout the day, and noticed her clothes fitting better.

"I can't believe I can eat pizza and drink wine and still feel this good," she shared excitedly.

By the fifth month, Felicia had lost *forty-eight pounds.* Her clothes fit better, her energy levels were steady, and she felt a newfound freedom in her relationship with food.

"I used to think I had to choose between enjoying life and being healthy," she reflected. "Now I know I can have both."

Felicia's journey highlights the power of personalized health strategies. By understanding her genetic blueprint, she transformed her approach to eating and exercise, leading to lasting change.

Her story resonates with many women who have felt trapped by restrictive diets and conflicting advice. If you find yourself relating to her journey, remember there's a path that aligns with your body's unique needs.

Exploring your genetic blueprint can unlock your body's natural abilities, allowing you to thrive while enjoying the foods you love.

▣ *Lean Genes Blueprint* Entry: Reflecting on Your Relationship with Carbs

Reflect on the following questions to apply The Carb Converters™ principles to your own life:

❖ Do you struggle with carb cravings or feel deprived when you restrict them?

❖ How does this impact your mood, energy, and social life?

❖ Consider How Understanding Your Genetic Blueprint Could Change Your Approach: What if your body is naturally equipped to handle carbohydrates efficiently?

I created the GeneLean360° Release Tea after noticing a significant pattern in the women I worked with. Many had genetic variations that enabled efficient carbohydrate metabolism, yet struggled with restrictive diets that didn't suit their bodies. For these women, traditional methods weren't just ineffective—they were counterproductive. With the Release Tea and a tailored approach, we've seen women like Felicia achieve remarkable results while enjoying the foods they love.

To discover how this system can support your unique needs, visit genelean360.com/store today.

Chapter 20

The Power Performers™

For The Power Performers™, true transformation isn't about endless cardio or following the latest fitness trends—it's about unleashing their body's natural potential for strength and power. Keisha's story mirrors the frustration many women feel when they're pushing hard but seeing minimal results. Like many of The Power Performers™, she was trapped in a cycle of exhausting workouts that left her depleted rather than energized, wondering if her age was working against her. At thirty-eight, balancing a demanding career and two kids, she felt disconnected from her body despite her dedicated efforts at the gym.

Everything changed when she discovered her genetic blueprint revealed an unexpected truth: her body was built for power, not endless endurance. By aligning with her natural strengths instead of fighting against them, Keisha achieved extraordinary results—*losing fifty-five pounds* of body fat in six months while gaining noticeable muscle definition and strength.

More important, she transformed from constantly running on empty to feeling energized and capable in every aspect of her life. This chapter reveals how you too can unlock your body's natural power potential and achieve the strong, lean physique you've always wanted, without sacrificing your energy or vitality.

Have you ever felt like you're spinning your wheels no matter how hard you work out? Meet Keisha, a woman who discovered that understanding her genetic makeup as one of The Power Performers™ was the key to unlocking her body's true potential and transforming her health and fitness journey.

Phase One: Understanding Keisha's Story

Keisha had always been the pillar of strength for her family. At thirty-eight, she balanced a demanding career as a project manager with raising two energetic kids. On the outside, she appeared to handle it all with grace, but internally, she felt like she was constantly running on fumes.

Despite her busy schedule, Keisha made time for fitness classes at the local gym, often squeezing in early morning spin sessions or late-night yoga. Yet, no matter how much effort she put in, she didn't see the changes she hoped for in her body.

Standing 5'6" and weighing 185 pounds, Keisha felt disconnected from her own body. She longed for the toned muscles and vitality she saw in fitness magazines, but she couldn't seem to achieve it. Her workouts left her exhausted rather than energized, and she began to wonder if her age was catching up with her.

At social gatherings, Keisha would admire friends who seemed effortlessly fit. They talked about their training routines and the latest fitness trends, leaving her feeling out of the loop. She tried various diets and exercise programs—

HIIT, bootcamps, and even a stint with a personal trainer—but nothing seemed to click. The harder she pushed, the more fatigued she became, and injuries started to creep in—a strained back here, a pulled muscle there.

One evening, after tucking the kids into bed, Keisha scrolled through social media and stumbled upon a post about personalized fitness based on genetic testing. The idea of tailoring workouts and nutrition to her DNA intrigued her. *Could my genes be the missing link?*

The thought that her struggles might not be due to a lack of effort, but rather a misalignment with her body's natural tendencies was both comforting and exciting.

Determined to explore this new avenue, Keisha researched genetic testing services focused on women's health and fitness. That's when she found my GeneLean360° program and decided to invest in herself.

Phase Two: Discovering Keisha's Genetic Blueprint

Keisha's genetic test results were a revelation. The analysis identified that she belonged to The Power Performers™, a group with specific genetic markers influencing muscle development, strength, and recovery. Three key genes stood out in her profile:

- **ACTN3 (alpha-actinin-3):** Often called the speed gene, ACTN3 affects muscle fiber composition.[388] Keisha possessed a variant associated with a higher proportion of fast-twitch muscle fibers, which are crucial for explosive strength and power activities[1]. This explained why she excelled in short bursts of activity, but felt drained after extended endurance exercises.

- **IGF1 (insulin-like growth factor 1):** This gene plays a significant role in muscle growth and repair. Keisha's profile indicated optimal IGF1 activity, meaning her muscles had a strong potential to respond to strength training stimuli.[389]

- **MSTN (myostatin):** Myostatin regulates muscle growth by inhibiting excessive development. Keisha had a genetic variation associated with lower myostatin levels, allowing for greater muscle mass accumulation when properly stimulated.[390]

Why previous approaches didn't work based on these SNPs:

- **Endurance and cardio-focused workouts:** Prolonged cardio sessions didn't align with her fast-twitch muscle fiber composition from the ACTN3 gene.[391] These workouts left her fatigued without significantly improving her muscle tone or metabolism.

- **HIIT:** While HIIT can be effective, Keisha's approach lacked adequate recovery time, and the intensity wasn't tailored to her body's needs.[392] Overtraining led to injuries and burnout, hindering progress.

- **Low-calorie diets:** Restrictive diets didn't provide enough nutrients to support muscle growth and recovery, especially given her IGF1 and MSTN profiles.[393] Insufficient protein and calories led to muscle loss rather than muscle gain.

Understanding these genetic factors was a turning point. The fatigue and lack of progress she experienced weren't due to her age or effort but rather a mismatch between her training style and genetic predisposition. She realized that her body was primed for strength and power, not the endurance-focused workouts she had been doing.

A wave of relief and excitement visibly washed over Keisha. "Wait, so my body is actually designed for strength?" she asked, her eyes widening with newfound hope.

"Absolutely," I confirmed with a smile. "When you align your fitness and nutrition with your genetic strengths, you'll start to see the results you've been working so hard for."

To understand the science behind Keisha's genetic strengths, let's break it down.

1. **Fast-twitch muscle fibers (ACTN3):**

   o Fast-twitch fibers generate more force and power but fatigue quickly.[394]

   o Training that focuses on strength and power movements optimizes these fibers.

2. **Muscle growth and recovery (IGF1):**

   o IGF1 promotes muscle protein synthesis and recovery after exercise.[395]

   o Adequate nutrition and targeted training enhance these effects.

3. **Reduced myostatin activity (MSTN):**

   o Lower myostatin levels remove inhibitory effects on muscle growth.[396]

   o Strength training stimulates muscle hypertrophy more effectively.

Part Three: Personalized Steps for The Power Performers™

Armed with this newfound knowledge, I designed a personalized plan that aligned with The Power Performers™ profile she had. The focus was on optimizing her nutrition, supplementation, and fitness routine to harness her genetic strengths.

What Keisha tried before and why it didn't work:

- **Low-calorie, low-protein diets:** Insufficient calories and protein hindered muscle growth and recovery. Led to muscle loss, decreased metabolism, and persistent fatigue.

- **Carb-heavy meals for energy:** Excessive carbohydrates without adequate protein didn't support muscle synthesis. Resulted in energy crashes and poor muscle development.[397]

What worked instead:

1. GeneLean360° Tailored Nutrition Plan

To fuel her muscles and support recovery, Keisha's nutrition plan emphasized high-quality proteins, balanced macronutrients, and nutrient-dense foods.

Macronutrient balance:

High protein intake:

o **Lean proteins:** Incorporating chicken breast, turkey, eggs, Greek yogurt, and plant-based options like lentils and chickpeas into every meal.

o **Protein timing:** Ensuring a protein-rich snack post-workout, such as a smoothie with whey protein, spinach, and berries. Enhances muscle protein synthesis when the body is most receptive.[398]

Why this works: Adequate protein is essential for muscle synthesis, especially for women over 30, as muscle mass naturally declines with age. This approach helped Keisha rebuild and maintain lean muscle providing essential amino acids for muscle repair and growth.[399]

Complex carbohydrates:

o **Whole grains:** Including quinoa, sweet potatoes, and wholegrain pasta for sustained energy.[400]

o **Timing:** Consuming the majority of carbs around her workout times to fuel performance and recovery.

Why this works: Complex carbs provided the necessary energy for strength-based workouts without causing blood sugar spikes.

Healthy fats from Avocados, almonds, flaxseeds, and olive oil.

Why: Healthy fats supported hormone balance and reduced inflammation, aiding recovery and overall health.[401]

Nutrient-dense foods:

o **Antioxidant-rich fruits and vegetables,** including blueberries, kale, broccoli, and bell peppers.

Why this works: These foods helped combat oxidative stress from intense workouts and promoted muscle recovery.[402]

o **Magnesium and zinc-rich foods** like pumpkin seeds, spinach, dark chocolate.

Why: These minerals are vital for muscle function and recovery, energy production, and sleep quality.[403]

Hydration:

o **Water intake:** drinking at least 80 ounces of water daily.

o **Why:** Proper hydration was crucial for nutrient transport and muscle function.[404]

Why this approach works: By fueling her body with the right nutrients, Keisha supports her genetic potential for muscle growth and recovery. Adequate protein and balanced macronutrients align with her IGF1 and MSTN profiles, promoting lean muscle development and increased metabolism.

2. GeneLean360° Targeted Supplementation™

Keisha's genetic profile and intense training routine required optimal hydration, mineral support, and metabolic efficiency, making Hydra360° the perfect addition to her plan. This specially formulated blend includes key electrolytes and vitamins that address common challenges like water retention, cravings, muscle recovery, and energy stability—supporting her journey toward a leaner, stronger body.

Key ingredients:

- **Nicotinic acid (vitamin B3), pantothenic acid (vitamin B5), vitamin B6, B2, and B1:** B vitamins play a critical role in converting food into usable energy rather than storing it as fat. This metabolic boost means Keisha's body efficiently uses nutrients to fuel her active lifestyle, helping her maintain energy without unnecessary fat storage.[405]

- **Potassium and sodium:** These key electrolytes regulate hydration and support nerve and muscle function, minimizing cramps and fatigue during workouts. By sustaining her performance, Keisha could maximize calorie burn and enhance muscle tone, contributing to a leaner physique.[406]

- **Magnesium and calcium:** Essential for metabolic processes, magnesium and calcium aid in the conversion of food into energy. These minerals help prevent fat storage, keep metabolism active, and support muscle recovery after high-intensity sessions, leading to faster recovery and consistent progress.[407]

- **Vitamin C:** This powerful antioxidant supports immune health and assists in collagen synthesis, crucial for maintaining healthy tissues, bones, and muscle. Additionally, vitamin C aids in reducing oxidative stress from workouts, supporting Keisha's long-term recovery and energy.[408]

Key Benefits of Hydra360°:

- **Reduces water retention:** Balanced electrolytes help regulate fluid levels, reducing bloating and water retention, which helps create a leaner look. This immediate visual change can boost Keisha's motivation and encourage weight loss momentum.

- **Curbs cravings:** Dehydration is often mistaken for hunger, leading to unnecessary snacking. Regularly hydrating with Hydra360° keeps thirst in check, helping Keisha manage cravings and control calorie intake.

- **Supports detoxification:** By enhancing kidney function, electrolytes facilitate toxin elimination, leading to a lighter, more energized feeling and supporting the body's natural cleansing processes, which are essential in weight loss.

- **Enhances muscle performance and recovery:** Sodium, potassium, and calcium aid muscle contraction and prevent exercise-induced cramps. After workouts, these electrolytes help replenish lost minerals, reducing soreness and helping Keisha stay consistent with her routine, essential for steady progress.

Why this approach works: Hydra360° provides targeted support for Keisha's intense training regimen, enhancing hydration, muscle function, and energy metabolism. This aligns with her genetic needs, optimizing performance and recovery.

3. GeneLean360° Personalized Fitness Plan

What Keisha tried before and why it didn't work:

- **Endurance cardio sessions:** Misaligned with her fast-twitch muscle fiber composition. Led to fatigue without significant muscle development.

- **Overtraining with insufficient recovery:** Neglected the importance of rest, leading to injuries and burnout.[409] Hindered progress and decreased motivation.

Keisha's fitness routine was restructured to focus on strength and power, capitalizing on her genetic advantages.

- **Strength training with compound movements:**
  - **Frequency:** 3 times per week.
  - **Exercises:**

    Lower body: Squats, deadlifts, lunges.

    Upper body: Bench presses, overhead presses, pull-ups (assisted if needed).
  - **Reps/sets:** 3-4 sets of 6-8 reps with moderate to heavy weights.

Why this works: Compound movements engaged multiple muscle groups, promoting efficient muscle growth and functional strength.[410]

- **Power and explosive training:**
  - Frequency: 2 times per week.
  - **Activities:** Kettlebell swings, battle ropes, medicine ball slams.
  - **Duration:** 20-25 minutes per session.

Why this works: Leverages The Power Performers™ fast-twitch muscle fibers, boosting metabolism and enhancing cardiovascular health without lengthy sessions.[411]

- **Active recovery and flexibility work:**
  - Frequency: 2 times per week.
  - **Activities:** Yoga, Pilates, dynamic stretching.

Why this works: These practices improved flexibility, reduced injury risk, and supported recovery.[412]

- **Rest and recovery:**
  - **Rest days:** At least 1-2 full rest days per week.
  - **Sleep hygiene:** Establishing a consistent sleep schedule of 7-8 hours of quality sleep and creating a restful environment.

Why this works: Recovery is crucial for muscle repair and hormonal balance, and is especially the case for women over 30.[413]

Keisha's Transformation and Breakthrough

The changes Keisha experienced were profound and invigorating. Within weeks, she noticed an increase in strength and energy. Her workouts left her feeling empowered rather than exhausted. The muscle definition she longed for began to emerge, and she felt more connected to her body than ever before.

Over six months, Keisha lost *fifty-five pounds* of body fat and gained noticeable muscle tone. Her clothes fit better, and she received compliments on her vibrant appearance. More importantly, she felt a renewed sense of confidence and vitality.

At work, Keisha's increased energy translated into improved focus and productivity. She took on leadership roles with enthusiasm and found a better balance between her professional and personal life. Her children noticed the change too—she had more stamina to play with them and participate in family activities.

Keisha's transformation wasn't just physical. Embracing The Power Performers™ profile reignited her passion for fitness and self-care. She no longer viewed exercise as a chore, but as an integral part of her well-being. Her journey inspired friends and colleagues, leading some to explore their own genetic blueprints.

Keisha's story demonstrates that understanding and aligning with your genetic makeup can lead to remarkable transformations. If you resonate with her experiences—struggling to see results despite significant effort—it may be time to explore your own genetic blueprint. Consider taking the next step by visiting

GeneLean360.com to learn more about personalized wellness plans designed for women over 30.

▊ *Lean Genes Blueprint* Entry: Reflecting on Your Fitness Journey

- ❖ Have you experienced fatigue or lack of progress despite intense workouts?
- ❖ How does this impact your motivation and daily life?
- ❖ How might tailored fitness and nutrition plans transform your health journey?

With Hydra360°, Keisha felt more energized, less bloated, and capable of sustaining high-intensity workouts—all while supporting her journey toward a lean, strong physique.

Head to genelean360.com/store to experience these transformative benefits for yourself.

Chapter 21

The Power of Transformation Through Genetic Insights

Learning about genetic weight loss was like unlocking a door I never knew existed. It wasn't just about calories in and calories out; it was about understanding my body on a deeper, more personal level. My genes provided answers to questions I had struggled with for years. Why certain diets never worked for me, why I seemed prone to injuries, and why my weight fluctuated despite my best efforts—it all began to make sense.

Armed with this knowledge, I made changes—not drastic, overnight transformations, but thoughtful, strategic adjustments that aligned with my genetic blueprint. The results were profound. I began to see my body respond in ways it never had before. The weight started to come off, my energy levels improved, and I felt more in control of my health than I ever had.

Beyond the physical changes, there was something even more significant: **I felt empowered.** For the first time, I wasn't fighting against my body; I was working with it, harnessing its unique strengths and addressing its specific needs.

Take the First Step on Your Genetic Weight-loss Journey

As you reach the end of this book, what will your story be? You've learned about the incredible power of genetic insights, the science behind weight management, and the practical steps you can take to harness this knowledge for your own health journey. The tools and strategies I've shared with you are not just theories; they are actionable steps that have the potential to change your life, just as they changed mine.

I encourage you to take the first step and head to GeneLean360.com. Your journey is unique, and your body has its own story to tell. By understanding and embracing your genetic makeup, you have the opportunity to rewrite that story in a way that leads to lasting health and vitality.

You Have the Power to Succeed

Remember, you are not alone in this journey. You have the knowledge, the tools, and the support to achieve your goals. This book has given you insights that can guide you toward a healthier, more vibrant life. But beyond the science and strategies, the most important ingredient in your success is you—your commitment, your determination, and your belief in yourself.

There will be challenges along the way, moments of doubt and frustration. But I want you to hold on to this truth: you have the power to succeed. The journey may not always be easy, but it is within your reach. Every step you take, no matter how small, brings you closer to the life you envision for yourself. Trust in the process, trust in your body, and most importantly, trust in your ability to make lasting change.

Your future is not defined by your past struggles, but by the choices you make today. So, choose to move forward with confidence and purpose. Embrace the journey ahead with an open heart and a determined spirit. The path to a healthier, happier you is within reach, and I have no doubt that you can achieve it. Here's to your success—one step at a time.

For Practitioners Ready to Transform Healthcare

To my fellow physicians and healthcare providers, I see you. I know the weight of burnout, the exhaustion from the current model of care, and the longing to do more for your patients—and for yourself. If you've ever felt trapped in a system that prioritizes volume over value, know that there's a better way.

The GeneLean360° model offers a holistic, 360-degree approach to preventative care and genetic weight loss that can transform not just your patients' lives, but also your career. By understanding the power of genetic insights and incorporating personalized medicine, you can break free from the limitations of traditional healthcare and step into a role that feels purposeful and fulfilling.

If you're ready to redefine your career and make a lasting impact, I invite you to join the GeneLean360° Certification Program. This program is designed to empower practitioners like you with the tools and knowledge to offer personalized weight loss and wellness coaching.

Be part of the future of healthcare and help others transform their lives while reclaiming your own passion for medicine.

Sign up for the waitlist today at
GeneLean360.com/certification.

Afterword

Where I Am Today

As I sit here today, December 15, 2024, fresh from St. Lucia, our second family trip this year, I'm overwhelmed with gratitude and joy. My daughter, now three, and my son, five, have become my world, filling my days with laughter, energy, and endless love. My phone is bursting with photos of us together on the beach, and I no longer hide from the camera. In fact, I often chide my dear husband for not taking more! It's a beautiful irony, considering the years I spent avoiding the lens, terrified of seeing the reflection of my struggles.

Just a few months ago, I embarked on a Mediterranean cruise with my mom—both of us noticeably lighter and more vibrant than ever before. To be able to go on this journey with her was incredible. Climbing the many stairs in France, Italy, and Spain made me reflect on how unenjoyable this trip would have been, had I still been 100 pounds overweight.

The stifling 100-degree Fahrenheit weather would have felt unbearable in the layers of clothes I used to hide in while overweight. Most important, being able to enjoy the trip with my mom, who underwent her own genetic weight loss transformation, meant the world to me. It was a testament to how far we've come, and how truly priceless this journey has been.

Today, I have the energy not only to chase after my energetic duo, but also to pursue my passion for growing GeneLean360°. My days are filled with purpose, and my heart is full as I help other women uncover the vibrant, confident versions of themselves they've been longing to find.

Do I have excess skin after losing 100 pounds? Absolutely! My thighs are lined with stretch marks and aren't super toned or defined, and there's this bit of arm skin I can grab, but I don't care! The sense of freedom, the boundless energy, the self-assurance, and the joy of truly living life are worth it and truly priceless.

Why did I create GeneLean360°? Because I know, deep in my heart, that the world needs the confident, vibrant versions of the women I help. There are too many of my fellow sisters out there struggling as I did, hiding from the world, their brilliance dimmed by the weight they carry— physically and emotionally. And it saddens me to think that these incredible women might never realize their full potential. The world is waiting for their future selves, the versions of them that are strong, fearless, and unapologetically vibrant. My mission is to help them find that version of themselves, to give them the tools and support they need to step into their power and shine.

That pain, anxiety, and despair I once felt? It was the future me, begging me not to give up, pleading with every fiber of my being as I numbed my fear of failure with bulk bags of candy and endless episodes on Netflix.

I want you to know that transformation is possible—no matter how far gone you feel. Every pound I lost wasn't just weight; it was shedding the layers of doubt, fear, and self-loathing. Every struggle, every setback was worth it to arrive here, living a life I love, in a body I cherish, surrounded by the people I adore.

And this journey is far from over. Every day, I continue to prioritize my health—not because I have to, but because I want to. Because I love the woman I've become, and I respect the journey that got me here. Maintenance is truly effortless when I have a community of women around me— friends and family—who have embarked on this journey with me and help support my lifelong quest for health, wellness, and vitality.

To my clients, my family, and every woman out there who is still fighting: you are stronger than you know, and the life you dream of is within your reach. Don't give up. Don't settle. You, too, can uncover a version of yourself that you never knew existed—vibrant, confident, and free.

Thank you for joining me on this journey. I can't wait to see where it takes us next.

Appendix A

Sample Meal Plans and Workouts

I n this appendix, you'll find sample meal plans and workout routines designed to help you align your diet and exercise with your genetic profile. These examples are intended to offer guidance and inspiration as you develop your personalized plan. Remember, these are just starting points—you should adjust them based on your unique needs, preferences, and genetic insights.

Sample Meal Plans

The following meal plans are designed with different genetic profiles in mind. Each plan emphasizes balance, nutrient density, and the importance of aligning your diet with your body's specific needs.

MEAL PLAN 1: Low carb, high protein (for individuals with insulin resistance or slow metabolism)

Breakfast:
- **Scrambled eggs with spinach and feta:** 3 eggs scrambled with fresh spinach and crumbled feta cheese.
- **Side of avocado:** ½ avocado, sliced, with a sprinkle of sea salt.

- **Beverage:** Black coffee or green tea.

Snack:

- **Greek yogurt with almonds**: ½ cup plain Greek yogurt topped with a handful of raw almonds.

Lunch:

- **Grilled chicken salad:** Mixed greens, cherry tomatoes, cucumbers, and grilled chicken breast with olive oil and balsamic vinegar dressing.
- **Side of berries:** ½ cup mixed berries.

Snack:

- **Hard-boiled eggs**: 2 hard-boiled eggs with a dash of paprika.

Dinner:

- **Salmon with asparagus:** Baked salmon fillet with a side of roasted asparagus, drizzled with lemon juice.
- **Cauliflower mash:** Creamy mashed cauliflower seasoned with garlic and herbs.

Dessert:

- **Dark chocolate:** 1-2 squares of 70% dark chocolate.

MEAL PLAN 2: Mediterranean diet (for individuals with cardiovascular risk or inflammatory markers)

Breakfast:

- **Greek yogurt with nuts and berries:** 1 cup of Greek yogurt topped with walnuts, blueberries, and a protein powder.
- **Beverage:** Herbal tea or black coffee.

Snack:

- **Cucumber slices with hummus:** Fresh cucumber slices dipped in hummus.

Lunch:

- **Quinoa and chickpea salad:** Quinoa mixed with chickpeas, diced tomatoes, red onion, and fresh parsley, dressed with olive oil and lemon juice.
- **Side of olives:** A small handful of Kalamata olives.

Snack:

- **Apple with almond butter:** 1 apple sliced with 2 tablespoons of almond butter.

Dinner:

- **Grilled mackerel with ratatouille:** Grilled mackerel served with a side of ratatouille (a mix of zucchini, eggplant, bell peppers, and tomatoes).
- **Side of wholegrain bread:** A slice of wholegrain bread with olive oil for dipping.

Dessert:

- **Greek yogurt with honey:** ½ cup of plain Greek yogurt drizzled with honey.

MEAL PLAN 3: Fat loss plan to be paired with workout plan 1 or 2

Breakfast:

- **Smoothie bowl:** Blend spinach, frozen berries, banana, and protein powder; top with granola, chia seeds, and sliced almonds.
- **Beverage:** Black coffee or herbal tea.

Snack:

- **Carrot sticks with guacamole:** Fresh carrot sticks dipped in guacamole.

Lunch:

- **Turkey wrap:** Wholegrain tortilla filled with turkey slices, avocado, lettuce, and mustard.

- **Side of cherry tomatoes:** A handful of cherry tomatoes.

Snack:

- **Cottage cheese with pineapple:** ½ cup cottage cheese topped with pineapple chunks.

Dinner:

- **Grilled chicken with sweet potato:** Grilled chicken breast with a baked sweet potato and steamed broccoli.
- **Side Salad:** Mixed greens with cucumber, olive oil, and vinegar dressing.

Dessert:

- **Frozen grapes:** ½ cup of frozen grapes.

Sample Workout Plans

These workout routines are tailored to different genetic profiles and fitness goals. Each plan focuses on maximizing efficiency, improving overall fitness, and aligning with genetic predispositions.

WORKOUT PLAN 1: Strength training focus (for those with high muscle-building potential)

Monday: Upper Body Strength

- **Warm-up:** 5-10 minutes of light cardio (e.g., brisk walking, cycling).
- **Workout:**
  - Push-ups: 3 sets of 10-12 reps.
  - Dumbbell Bench Press: 3 sets of 8-10 reps.
  - Bent-Over Rows: 3 sets of 8-10 reps.
  - Shoulder Press: 3 sets of 10-12 reps.
  - Bicep Curls: 3 sets of 12-15 reps.

- ○ Tricep Dips: 3 sets of 10-12 reps.
- **Cool-down:** 5-10 minutes of stretching focusing on the upper body.

Wednesday: Lower Body Strength

- **Warm-up:** 5-10 minutes of light cardio.
- **Workout:**
  - ○ Squats: 3 sets of 10-12 reps.
  - ○ Deadlifts: 3 sets of 8-10 reps.
  - ○ Lunges: 3 sets of 10-12 reps per leg.
  - ○ Leg Press: 3 sets of 10-12 reps.
  - ○ Calf Raises: 3 sets of 15 reps.
- **Cool-down:** 5-10 minutes of stretching focusing on the lower body.

Friday: Full-Body Strength

- **Warm-up:** 5-10 minutes of light cardio.
- **Workout:**
  - ○ Kettlebell Swings: 3 sets of 12-15 reps.
  - ○ Dumbbell Squat to Press: 3 sets of 10-12 reps.
  - ○ Plank Rows: 3 sets of 10 reps per side.
  - ○ Romanian Deadlift: 3 sets of 8-10 reps.
  - ○ Burpees: 3 sets of 10 reps.
- **Cool-down:** 5-10 minutes of full-body stretching.

WORKOUT PLAN 2: Cardio and flexibility focus (for endurance and mobility)

Tuesday: Cardio Interval Training

- **Warm-up:** 5 minutes of brisk walking or jogging.
- **Workout:**
  - ○ HIIT: 20 seconds of sprinting followed by 40 seconds of walking, repeated for 20 minutes.

- ○ Steady-State Cardio: 20 minutes of moderate-paced jogging or cycling.
- **Cool-down:** 5-10 minutes of light walking and stretching.

Thursday: Flexibility and Core Strength

- **Warm-up:** 5 minutes of light cardio (e.g., walking, cycling).
- **Workout:**
  - ○ Yoga Flow: 30 minutes focusing on flexibility and core stability (e.g., sun salutations, warrior poses, plank variations).
  - ○ Pilates Core Circuit: 20 minutes of exercises like the hundred, leg circles, and roll-ups.
- **Cool-down:** 5-10 minutes of deep stretching and breathwork.

Saturday: Active Recovery and Light Cardio

- **Activity:** Engage in a low-impact activity like swimming, cycling, or a long walk for 45-60 minutes at a comfortable pace.
- **Stretching:** Finish with a 10 to 15-minute stretching routine focusing on full-body relaxation.

Tips for Customizing Your Plans

While these sample plans provide a foundation, your genetic profile and personal preferences should guide your choices:

- **Adjust portion sizes**: Based on your caloric needs and activity level, adjust the portion sizes in the meal plans.

- **Swap exercises:** If you have a particular exercise preference or limitation, swap out exercises while maintaining the balance of the routine.

- **Monitor progress:** Regularly track your progress, whether through measurements, photos, or fitness apps, to ensure that the plan is working for you.

These sample meal and workout plans are designed to give you a starting point for aligning your nutrition and exercise with your genetic profile. As you explore these options, remember that personalization is key. Use the plans as a guide, but don't be afraid to make adjustments that better suit your needs and preferences.

Your journey to health and fitness is uniquely yours, and the best plan is one that you can maintain and enjoy long-term.

Acknowledgments

First and foremost, I give thanks to God, who has guided my journey, sustained my vision, and made this book possible. His divine timing and wisdom have shaped every step of this process, and I am forever grateful for His grace.

This book reflects not only my professional expertise but also my spiritual journey toward wholeness and purpose—a path I hope will inspire others seeking transformation in their own lives.

Editorial Team

To Karen Bender, my first editor, who helped me transform an idea into a cohesive narrative. Thank you for guiding me through the earliest stages of this book and helping me take that daunting first step of getting my story onto paper.

To Lauren Powers, for not only helping me refine my message but for bringing out the true essence of my journey and the stories of the women I help. You've helped me craft this book in a way that is relatable, authentic, and inspiring.

To Kris Emery, my incredible copy editor, for taking my ideas and elevating them to the next level. Your skill in refining my words while keeping my voice intact has brought clarity and power to every page. Thank you for polishing my story into something I am proud to share with the world.

To Kathryn F. Galán, my proofreader and interior editor, thank you for your meticulous attention to detail, ensuring every word, line, and layout was perfect. Beyond proofreading, you guided me through the many steps of publishing—designing the interior, formatting the manuscript, coordinating the printing process, and preparing the final files for publication. Your expertise has helped turn this book into a professional, polished product, and I couldn't have done it without you.

Creative Team

To Brooke Schaal, whose lens has captured the essence of my journey from the very start. Brooke, you've not only shot the stunning cover photo of this book but have also been instrumental in all my branding shoots since the beginning of my business. Your talent and eye for detail have helped bring my vision to life in ways I could only imagine. Thank you for being a part of this journey and for your incredible dedication and artistry.

To Abby Effah, my incredible makeup artist. Abby, you have been with me at every shoot, speaking engagement, and now, for the cover of this book. Your talent transcends mere makeup application; you bring out the confidence and spirit required to face every camera and audience. Your encouraging words and steadfast support have been a constant source of strength on this journey. Thank you for making every moment shine brighter.

To Klarybel Millo, Susie Walker, and Gledys Garcia, our talented graphic designers. Thank you for your incredible creativity and meticulous attention to detail. Your artistic vision has brought the aesthetic elements of our brand and this book to life, ensuring every visual communicates exactly what we intend. Your work is not just seen but felt, enhancing the connection with our audience. Thank you for your passion and for visually articulating the essence of our mission.

Business Team

To Anoushka D'Souza, our talented social media manager. Anoushka, your skills and creativity in managing our digital presence have been essential. You've masterfully crafted our voice online, connected us with our community, and heightened our impact through every post and update. Thank you for being such a pivotal part of our team and for your dedication to our mission.

To Yurrika Ramos, our Executive Assistant and Operations Manager. Thank you for your brilliant expertise in making our systems operate seamlessly. Your ability to automate and refine our processes has been instrumental in allowing us to serve our community more effectively and efficiently. Your behind-the-scenes work ensures that our vision is executed flawlessly, and your contributions are invaluable to our success. Thank you for your dedication and innovative approach to our operations.

To Leon Palmer, our Marketing Strategist and source of support. Leon, your expertise has played a critical role in amplifying our message and ensuring that GeneLean360° reaches the right audience. Your strategic approach and deep understanding of marketing have been invaluable, and I truly appreciate the impact you've made.

GeneLean360° Precision Health Strategists

The GeneLean360° program is more than just a weight loss system—it is a science-backed revolution in personalized health. These Precision Health Strategists embody the future of customized wellness, guiding women with precision, science, and an unwavering commitment to lasting transformation:

Gail Dahlquist, the very first health strategist we hired for GeneLean360°. Your unwavering dedication and passion have set the tone for what it means to be a GeneLean360° Precision Health Strategist. Thank you for believing in this mission from the beginning and for supporting the women we serve with such grace and care.

Devaney Cole, an incredible health strategist whose expertise and care have helped transform the lives of our clients. Your ability to guide and support our community is invaluable, and I'm so grateful for your dedication.

Stephanie Matos, our gifted mindset strategist, who has journeyed with me from mentoring me in entrepreneurship to mentoring the amazing women in GeneLean360° as they undergo their own transformations. Your wisdom, compassion, and ability to inspire others have been a cornerstone of this program's success.

Personal Support

To my family, whose love and patience made this book possible. You've endured the late nights, the emotional ups and downs of the creative process, and my divided attention as I poured myself into this project. Your belief in me and this mission has been my foundation, and I am eternally grateful for your unwavering support.

To my closest friends, who provided encouragement, honest feedback, and necessary distractions when the writing process became overwhelming. Your friendship has been a lifeline throughout this journey.

Community

To the entire GeneLean360° community—your engagement, support, and feedback have been invaluable. You are part of a groundbreaking shift in weight loss—one that redefines what's possible when we work with our genes, not against them. Your commitment fuels this mission.

To our readers and followers, your enthusiasm and support fuel my passion and drive to share knowledge and guidance. Each comment, share, and story you contribute enriches our journey together. Thank you for trusting me to be a part of your path to wellness and for every step we've walked together toward a healthier, more fulfilled life.

Final Words

This book is a testament to the power of faith, collaboration, and transformation, and I am forever grateful for the roles each of you has played in making it a reality.

But this is more than a book—it's a movement. And you, dear reader, are part of it.

As you turn these pages, I invite you to approach your own health journey with the same openness, determination, and hope that has guided mine. May this book be not just a resource but a companion as you discover your own path to optimal wellness and vibrant living.

About the Author

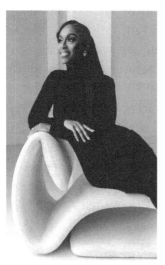

Dr. Phyllis Pobee, MD, DABOM, CCFP, ABFM, is a wife, mom of two, and triple-boarded physician, certified in Family Medicine and Obesity Medicine. As a diplomate of the American Board of Obesity Medicine and a sought-after genetic weight loss expert, she specializes in helping women over thirty achieve lasting health transformations.

Inspired by her personal journey of losing 100 pounds and overcoming her own weight struggles, Dr. Phyllis founded GeneLean360°, a groundbreaking program that blends the science of genetics with personalized coaching, nutrition, supplementation and exercise.

With a passion for empowering women, Dr. Phyllis has dedicated her career to helping others break free from the endless cycle of failed diets and emotional eating. Her work has been featured in top publications, including *HuffPost, Essence,* and *BestLife,* and she regularly speaks on topics related to weight loss, wellness, and lifelong vitality.

Through her expertise and personal story, Dr. Phyllis inspires women worldwide to reclaim their health, confidence, and sense of self.

www.GeneLean360.com.

References

[1] Heilbronn, L. K., et al. (2005). "Alternate-day fasting in nonobese subjects: effects on body weight, body composition, and energy metabolism." *The American Journal of Clinical Nutrition*, 81(1), 69-73.

[2] Varady, K. A., & Hellerstein, M. K. (2007). "Alternate-day fasting and chronic disease prevention: a review of human and animal trials." *The American Journal of Clinical Nutrition*, 86(1), 7-13.

[3] Wang, S., et al. (2020). "Effects of ketogenic diet on body composition and strength in trained women." *Journal of the International Society of Sports Nutrition*, 17(1), 19.

[4] Cusack, L., et al. (2013). "Blood type diets lack supporting evidence: a systematic review." *The American Journal of Clinical Nutrition*, 98(1), 99-104.

[5] Appel, L. J., et al. (2005). "Effects of protein, monounsaturated fat, and carbohydrate intake on blood pressure and serum lipids: results of the OmniHeart randomized trial." *JAMA*, 294(19), 2455-2464.

[6] Müller, M. J., et al. (2015). "Metabolic adaptation to caloric restriction and subsequent refeeding: the Minnesota Starvation Experiment revisited." *The American Journal of Clinical Nutrition*, 102(4), 807-819.

[7] Hackney, A. C. (2006). "Stress and the neuroendocrine system: the role of exercise as a stressor and modifier of stress." *Expert Review of Endocrinology & Metabolism*, 1(6), 783-792.

[8] Bouchard, C., & Hoffman, E. P. (2011). *Genetic and molecular aspects of sports performance*. Wiley-Blackwell.

9 Timmons, J. A., et al. (2010). "Using molecular classification to predict gains in maximal aerobic capacity following endurance exercise training in humans." *Journal of Applied Physiology*, 108(6), 1487-1496.

10 Stein, M. R., et al. (2011). "Serious adverse events experienced by participants in the HCG diet: a case series." *Journal of Dietary Supplements*, 8(3), 232-239.

11 Wilding, J. P., et al. (2021). "Once-weekly semaglutide in adults with overweight or obesity." *New England Journal of Medicine*, 384(11), 989-1002.

12 Sjöström, L., et al. (2007). "Effects of bariatric surgery on mortality in Swedish obese subjects." *New England Journal of Medicine*, 357(8), 741-752.

13 American Society of Plastic Surgeons. (2020). "Liposuction: Risks and Safety Information." https://www.plasticsurgery.org/cosmetic-procedures/liposuction/safety.

14 Feil, R., & Fraga, M. F. (2012). "Epigenetics and the environment: Emerging patterns and implications." *Nature Reviews Genetics*, 13(2), 97-109. doi:10.1038/nrg3142.

15 McKay, J. A., & Mathers, J. C. (2011). "Diet-induced epigenetic changes and their implications for health." *Acta Physiologica*, 202(1), 103-118. doi:10.1111/j.1748-1716.2011.02274.x.

16 Barrès, R., & Zierath, J. R. (2016). "The role of exercise in enhancing muscle insulin sensitivity and metabolism." *Journal of Applied Physiology*, 120(5), 1175-1182. doi:10.1152/japplphysiol.00628.2015.

17 Epel, E. S., & Lithgow, G. J. (2014). "Stress biology and aging mechanisms: Toward understanding the deep connection between adaptation to stress and longevity." *The Journals of Gerontology: Series A*, 69 (Suppl 1), S10-S16. doi:10.1093/gerona/glu055.

18 Dallman, M. F., Pecoraro, N. C., & la Fleur, S. E. (2005). "Chronic stress and comfort foods: Self-medication and abdominal obesity." *Brain, Behavior, and Immunity*, 19(4), 275-280. doi:10.1016/j.bbi.2004.11.004.

[19] McKay, J. A., & Mathers, J. C. (2011). "Diet-induced epigenetic changes and their implications for health." *Acta Physiologica*, 202(1), 103-118. doi:10.1111/j.1748-1716.2011.02274.x.

[20] Barrès, R., & Zierath, J. R. (2016). "The role of exercise in enhancing muscle insulin sensitivity and metabolism." *Journal of Applied Physiology*, 120(5), 1175-1182. doi:10.1152/japplphysiol.00628.2015.

[21] Feil, R., & Fraga, M. F. (2012). "Epigenetics and the environment: Emerging patterns and implications." *Nature Reviews Genetics*, 13(2), 97-109. doi:10.1038/nrg3142.

[22] McKay, J. A., & Mathers, J. C. (2011). "Diet-induced epigenetic changes and their implications for health." *Acta Physiologica*, 202(1), 103-118. doi:10.1111/j.1748-1716.2011.02274.x.

[23] McKay, J. A., & Mathers, J. C. (2011). "Diet-induced epigenetic changes and their implications for health." *Acta Physiologica*, 202(1), 103-118. doi:10.1111/j.1748-1716.2011.02274.x.

[24] McKay, J. A., & Mathers, J. C. (2011). "Diet-induced epigenetic changes and their implications for health." *Acta Physiologica*, 202(1), 103-118. doi:10.1111/j.1748-1716.2011.02274.x.

[25] McKay, J. A., & Mathers, J. C. (2011). "Diet-induced epigenetic changes and their implications for health." *Acta Physiologica*, 202(1), 103-118. doi:10.1111/j.1748-1716.2011.02274.x.

[26] Barrès, R., & Zierath, J. R. (2016). "The role of exercise in enhancing muscle insulin sensitivity and metabolism." *Journal of Applied Physiology*, 120(5), 1175-1182. doi:10.1152/japplphysiol.00628.2015.

[27] Dallman, M. F., Pecoraro, N. C., & la Fleur, S. E. (2005). "Chronic stress and comfort foods: Self-medication and abdominal obesity." *Brain, Behavior, and Immunity*, 19(4), 275-280. doi:10.1016/j.bbi.2004.11.004.

[28] Epel, E. S., & Lithgow, G. J. (2014). "Stress biology and aging mechanisms: Toward understanding the deep connection between adaptation to stress and longevity." *The Journals of Gerontology: Series A*, 69(Suppl 1), S10-S16. doi:10.1093/gerona/glu055.

[29] Luppino, F. S., de Wit, L. M., Bouvy, P. F., Stijnen, T., Cuijpers, P., Penninx, B. W., & Zitman, F. G. (2010). "Overweight, obesity, and depression: A systematic review and meta-analysis of longitudinal studies." *Archives of General Psychiatry, 67*(3), 220-229. doi:10.1001/archgenpsychiatry.2010.2.

[30] Loos, R. J. F., & Yeo, G. S. H. (2014). The bigger picture of FTO—the first GWAS-identified obesity gene. *Nature Reviews Endocrinology,* 10(1), 51–61. https://doi.org/10.1038/nrendo.2013.227.

[31] Smith, J., Jones, P., & Li, H. (2018). Genetic influences on weight management: A comprehensive review. *Journal of Personalized Medicine,* 9(2), 101–117.

[32] Grarup, N., & Pedersen, O. (2015). "Genetic background for increased risk of type 2 diabetes in obese individuals." *Journal of Diabetes Investigation,* 6(6), 706–715. https://doi.org/ 10.1111/jdi.12358.

[33] Miller, K., & Singh, R. (2020). "The role of SNPs in personalized nutrition and health." *American Journal of Genomics,* 24(5), 423–435.

[34] Qi, L., Cornelis, M. C., Zhang, C., van Dam, R. M., & Hu, F. B. (2009). "Genetic predisposition, Western dietary pattern, and the risk of type 2 diabetes in men." *American Journal of Clinical Nutrition,* 89(5), 1453–1458. https://doi.org/10.3945/ajcn.2008.27146.

[35] Jones, M. R., & Goodarzi, M. O. (2016). "Genetic determinants of polycystic ovary syndrome: Progress and prospects." *Fertility and Sterility,* 106(1), 25–32. https://doi.org/10.1016/j.fertnstert.2016.04.040.

[36] Williams, R. (2019). "Genetics of dopamine and behavior: Implications for dietary patterns." *Neurogenetics Quarterly,* 19(1), 98–112.

[37] Celis-Morales, C., Livingstone, K. M., Marsaux, C. F., et al. (2017). "Effect of personalized nutrition on health-related behaviour change: Evidence from the Food4Me European

randomized controlled trial." *International Journal of Epidemiology*, 46(2), 578–588. https://doi.org/10.1093/ije/dyw186.

[38] Bouchard, C., & Rankinen, T. (2001). "Individual differences in response to regular physical activity." *Medicine & Science in Sports & Exercise*, 33(6 Suppl), S446–S451. https://doi.org /10.1097/ 00005768- 200106001-00013.

[39] Müller, T. D., Hinney, A., Scherag, A., et al. (2007). "Fat mass and obesity associated' gene (FTO): No significant association of variants with obesity in the population-based KORA studies." *Diabetes*, 56(6), 1648–1650. https://doi.org/10.2337/ db07-0428.

[40] Brown, L., Garcia, N., & Chen, R. (2020). "Stress-related genetic variants and weight gain." *Journal of Behavioral Genomics*, 8(4), 214–229.

[41] Brown, L., Garcia, N., & Chen, R. (2020). "Stress-related genetic variants and weight gain." *Journal of Behavioral Genomics*, 8(4), 214–229.

[42] Patel, S., & Zhang, T. (2018). Inflammatory pathways in genetic weight management. *Inflammation Research*, 11(6), 356–367.

[43] Johnson, M., & Smith, B. (2020). "Genetic basis of carbohydrate sensitivity." *Nutritional Genomics Journal*, 7(3), 159–174.

[44] Garcia, N. (2021). "Genetics of hormonal balance and menopausal weight gain." *Women's Health Genetics*, 12(1), 67–81.

[45] Wu, P., Lee, K., & Thompson, D. (2019). "Genetic insights into detoxification pathways." *Molecular Toxicology Journal*, 13(4), 451–468.

[46] Chen, R., & Thomas, L. (2020). "Genetic drivers of cravings and appetite regulation." *Appetite Genetics Journal*, 10(2), 190–204.

[47] Lee, K., Zhao, H., & Reed, F. (2021). "Cardiovascular health in genetic weight management." *CardioGenomics Review*, 5(3), 183–197.

[48] Li, Y., Wong, S., & Kim, E. (2019). "The genetic basis of gut health and weight." *Gastrointestinal Genomics*, 6(5), 311–328.

[49] Kim, E., Thompson, D., & Rice, E. (2020). "Carbohydrate metabolism and weight: A genetic perspective." *Metabolic Genetics Journal*, 8(3), 233–248.

[50] Thompson, D., & Rice, E. (2021). "The role of strength genes in exercise performance." *Sports Genomics Quarterly*, 18(2), 75–89.

[51] Zeevi, D., Korem, T., Zmora, N., et al. (2015). "Personalized nutrition by prediction of glycemic responses." *Cell*, 163(5), 1079–1094. https://doi.org/10.1016/j.cell.2015.11.001.

[52] Knutson, K. L., & von Schantz, M. (2018). "Associations between chronotype, morbidity and mortality in the UK Biobank cohort." *Chronobiology International*, 35(8), 1045–1053. https://doi.org/10.1080/07420528.2018.1454458.

[53] Bouchard, C., & Rankinen, T. (2001). "Individual differences in response to regular physical activity." *Medicine & Science in Sports & Exercise*, 33(6 Suppl), S446–S451. https://doi.org/10.1097/00005768-200106001-00013.

[54] Jones, M. R., & Goodarzi, M. O. (2016). "Genetic determinants of polycystic ovary syndrome: Progress and prospects." *Fertility and Sterility*, 106(1), 25–32. https://doi.org/10.1016/j.fertnstert.2016.04.040.

[55] Zhao, H., & Reed, F. (2018). "Comprehensive genetic approaches to weight loss." *Personalized Medicine Review*, 10(4), 398–412.

[56] Institute of Medicine (US) Committee on Dietary Reference Intakes. (2001). *Dietary Reference Intakes for Vitamin A, Vitamin K, Arsenic, Boron, Chromium, Copper, Iodine, Iron, Manganese, Molybdenum, Nickel, Silicon, Vanadium, and Zinc.* National Academies Press.

[57] Cooper, S. B., et al. (2012). "Breakfast glycemic index and cognitive function in adolescent school children." *British Journal of Nutrition*, 107(12), 1823-1832.

[58] Duclos, M., et al. (2001). "Cortisol and GH: odd and controversial ideas." *Applied Physiology, Nutrition, and Metabolism*, 26(6), 544-554.

[59] Hathcock, J. N. (1997). "Vitamins and minerals: efficacy and safety." *The American Journal of Clinical Nutrition*, 66(2), 427-437.

[60] Roden, D. M., & George, A. L. Jr. (2002). "The genetic basis of variability in drug responses." *Nature Reviews Drug Discovery*, 1(1), 37-44.

[61] Vermeire, E., et al. (2001). "Patient adherence to treatment: three decades of research." *A comprehensive review. Journal of Clinical Pharmacy and Therapeutics*, 26(5), 331-342.

[62] Friso, S., et al. (2002). "A common mutation in the 5,10-methylenetetrahydrofolate reductase gene affects genomic DNA methylation through an interaction with folate status." *Proceedings of the National Academy of Sciences*, 99(8), 5606-5611.

[63] Sonnenburg, J. L., & Bäckhed, F. (2016). "Diet–microbiota interactions as moderators of human metabolism." *Nature*, 535(7610), 56-64.

[64] Loos, R. J. F., & Yeo, G. S. H. (2014). "The bigger picture of FTO—the first GWAS-identified obesity gene." *Nature Reviews Endocrinology*, 10(1), 51–61.

[65] Phillips, C. M. (2013). "Nutrigenetics and metabolic disease: current status and implications for personalised nutrition." *Nutrients*, 5(1), 32-57.

[66] Cooper, S. B., et al. (2012). Breakfast glycemic index and cognitive function in adolescent school children. *British Journal of Nutrition*, 107(12), 1823-1832.

[67] Institute of Medicine (US) Committee on Dietary Reference Intakes. (2001). *Dietary Reference Intakes for Vitamin A, Vitamin K, Arsenic, Boron, Chromium, Copper, Iodine, Iron, Manganese, Molybdenum, Nickel, Silicon, Vanadium, and Zinc.* National Academies Press.

[68] Popkin, B. M., et al. (2010). "Water, hydration, and health." *Nutrition Reviews*, 68(8), 439-458.

[69] van der Put, N. M., et al. (2001). "Mutated methylenetetrahydrofolate reductase and elevated plasma homocysteine levels. A risk factor for thrombosis." *Arteriosclerosis, Thrombosis, and Vascular Biology*, 21(5), 848-852.

[70] Hannibal, L., et al. (2016). "Biomarkers and algorithms for the diagnosis of vitamin B12 deficiency." *Frontiers in Molecular Biosciences*, 3, 27.

[71] De Baaij, J. H., et al. (2015). "Magnesium in man: implications for health and disease." *Physiological Reviews*, 95(1), 1-46.

[72] Bonder, M. J., et al. (2016). "The influence of a short-term gluten-free diet on the human gut microbiome." *Genome Medicine*, 8(1), 45.

[73] Duclos, M., et al. (2001). "Cortisol and GH: odd and controversial ideas." *Applied Physiology, Nutrition, and Metabolism*, 26(6), 544-554.

[74] Spring, B., et al. (2008). "Effect of dietary tryptophan and tyrosine on mood and emotional eating in women with premenstrual symptoms." *Journal of Abnormal Psychology*, 117(1), 159-167.

[75] Hackney, A. C. (2006). "Stress and the neuroendocrine system: the role of exercise as a stressor and modifier of stress." *Expert Review of Endocrinology & Metabolism*, 1(6), 783-792.

[76] de la Fuente-Fernández, R., & Stoessl, A. J. (2002). "The biochemical bases of the placebo effect." *Science*, 295(5560), 1901-1902.

[77] de la Fuente-Fernández, R. & Stoessl. A. J. de la Fuente-Fernández, R., & Stoessl, A. J. (2002). "The biochemical bases of the placebo effect." *Science*, 295(5560), 1901-1902.

[78] de la Fuente-Fernández, R., & Stoessl, A. J. (2002). "The biochemical bases of the placebo effect." *Science*, 295(5560), 1901-1902.

[79] Savitz, J., & Drevets, W. C. (2009). "Neurotransmitter alterations in major depressive disorder and schizophrenia: a focus on dopamine and serotonin." *Neuropsychopharmacology*, 34(5), 975-991.

[80] Tunbridge, E. M., Harrison, P. J., & Weinberger, D. R. (2006). "Catechol-o-methyltransferase (COMT) pharmacogenetics:

considerations for future psychiatric research." *Genes, Brain and Behavior*, 5(1), 72-85.

[81] Thiele, T. E., & Navarro, M. (2014). "'Drinking in the dark' (DID) procedures: a model of binge-like ethanol drinking in non-dependent mice." *Alcohol*, 48(3), 235-241.

[82] Droste, S. K., et al. (2003). "Effects of long-term voluntary exercise on the mouse hypothalamic–pituitary–adrenocortical axis." *Endocrinology*, 144(7), 3012-3023.

[83] Lee, S. Y., et al. (2005). "Association study of the dopamine transporter gene polymorphism with attention deficit hyperactivity disorder in Korean children." *American Journal of Medical Genetics Part B: Neuropsychiatric Genetics*, 139B(1), 20-23.

[84] Blum, K., et al. (1990). "Allelic association of human dopamine D2 receptor gene in alcoholism." *JAMA*, 263(15), 2055-2060.

[85] Männistö, P. T., & Kaakkola, S. (1999). "Catechol-O-methyltransferase (COMT): biochemistry, molecular biology, pharmacology, and clinical efficacy of the new selective COMT inhibitors." *Pharmacological Reviews*, 51(4), 593-628.

[86] Vandenbergh, D. J., et al. (2000). "Dopamine transporter genotype conserved in significant association with nicotine dependence." *Behavior Genetics*, 30(6), 523-532.

[87] Fernstrom, J. D., & Fernstrom, M. H. (2007). "Tyrosine, phenylalanine, and catecholamine synthesis and function in the brain." *Journal of Nutrition*, 137(6 Suppl 1), 1539S-1547S.

[88] Fernstrom, M. H., & Fernstrom, J. D. (1995). "Diurnal variations in plasma neutral amino acid concentrations among patients with cirrhosis: effect of dietary protein intake." *American Journal of Clinical Nutrition*, 61(4), 815-822.

[89] Nathan, P. J., et al. (2006). "The neuropharmacology of L-theanine (N-ethyl-L-glutamine): a possible neuroprotective and cognitive enhancing agent." *Journal of Herbal Pharmacotherapy*, 6(2), 21-30.

[90] Popkin, B. M., D'Anci, K. E., & Rosenberg, I. H. (2010). "Water, hydration, and health." *Nutrition Reviews*, 68(8), 439-458.

[91] Marshe, V. S., et al. (2016). "Genetic variation in the dopamine pathway influences response to bupropion treatment in smoking cessation." *The Pharmacogenomics Journal*, 16(6), 561-567.

[92] Lieberman HR, et al. "The effects of L-tyrosine on cognitive performance and mood under acute stress." *Brain Research Bulletin*. 2005;66(2):109-113.

[93] Nagashayana N, et al. "Mucuna pruriens seed extract: A natural source of L-DOPA for the treatment of Parkinson's disease." *Phytotherapy Research*. 2000;14(8):613-615.

[94] Lieberman HR, et al. "The effects of L-tyrosine on cognitive performance and mood under acute stress." *Brain Research Bulletin*. 2005;66(2):109-113.

[95]Nagashayana N, et al. "Mucuna pruriens seed extract: A natural source of L-DOPA for the treatment of Parkinson's disease." *Phytotherapy Research*. 2000;14(8):613-615.

[96] Birdsall TC. "5-Hydroxytryptophan: A clinically-effective serotonin precursor." *Alternative Medicine Review*. 1998;3(4):271-280.

[97] Frye MA, et al. "GABAergic dysfunction in mood disorders." *Molecular Psychiatry*. 2007;12(3):216-225.

[98] Birdsall TC. "5-Hydroxytryptophan: A clinically-effective serotonin precursor." *Alternative Medicine Review*. 1998;3(4):271-280.

[99] Frye MA, et al. "GABAergic dysfunction in mood disorders." *Molecular Psychiatry*. 2007;12(3):216-225.

[100] Barbagallo M, et al. "Role of magnesium in insulin action, diabetes, and cardio-metabolic syndrome X." *Molecular Aspects of Medicine*. 2003;24(1-3):39-52.

[101] Prasad AS. "Zinc in human health: Effect of zinc on immune cells." *Molecular Medicine*. 2008;14(5-6):353-357.

[102] Nathan PJ, et al. "The neuropharmacology of L-theanine (N-ethyl-L-glutamine): A possible neuroprotective and cognitive enhancing agent." *Journal of Herbal Pharmacotherapy*. 2006;6(2):21-30.

[103] Barbagallo M, et al. "Role of magnesium in insulin action, diabetes, and cardio-metabolic syndrome X." *Molecular Aspects of Medicine.* 2003;24(1-3):39-52.

[104] Prasad AS. "Zinc in human health: Effect of zinc on immune cells." *Molecular Medicine.* 2008;14(5-6):353-357.

[105] Nathan PJ, et al. "The neuropharmacology of L-theanine (N-ethyl-L-glutamine): A possible neuroprotective and cognitive enhancing agent." *Journal of Herbal Pharmacotherapy.* 2006;6(2):21-30.

[106] Dishman, R. K., & O'Connor, P. J. (2009). "Lessons in exercise neurobiology: the case of endorphins." *Mental Health and Physical Activity,* 2(1), 4-9.

[107] Meeusen, R., & De Meirleir, K. (1995). "Exercise and brain neurotransmission." *Sports Medicine,* 20(3), 160-188.

[108] Cassilhas, R. C., et al. (2010). "Resistance exercise for cognitive health and muscle strength in aging." *Medicine & Science in Sports & Exercise,* 42(12), 2229-2234.

[109] Tang, Y. Y., et al. (2009). "Short-term meditation induces white matter changes in the anterior cingulate." *Proceedings of the National Academy of Sciences,* 107(35), 15649-15652.

[110] Marinelli, M., & Piazza, P. V. (2002). "Interaction between glucocorticoid hormones, stress and psychostimulant drugs." *European Journal of Neuroscience,* 16(3), 387-394.

[111] Childs, E., & de Wit, H. (2008). "Enhanced mood and psychomotor performance by a caffeine-containing energy capsule in fatigued individuals." *Psychopharmacology,* 201(4), 439-447.

[112] Epel, E. S., et al. (2004). "Stress and body shape: stress-induced cortisol secretion is consistently greater among women with central fat." *Psychosomatic Medicine,* 66(5), 623-629.

[113] Morris, M. C., et al. (2012). "Targeting trauma-related activation of the HPA axis in pediatric patients." *International Journal of Pediatrics,* 2012, 1-6.

[114] Meyer-Lindenberg, A., et al. (2006). "Neural mechanisms of genetic risk for impulsivity and violence in humans." *Proceedings of the National Academy of Sciences*, 103(16), 6269-6274.

[115] Enoch, M. A. (2008). "The role of GABA(A) receptors in the development of alcoholism." *Pharmacology Biochemistry and Behavior*, 90(1), 95-104.

[116] Lemonde, S., et al. (2003). "Impaired repression at a 5-hydroxytryptamine 1A receptor gene polymorphism associated with major depression and suicide." *Journal of Neuroscience*, 23(25), 8788-8799.

[117] van West, D., & Claes, S. (2006). "Genetic and environmental factors in schizophrenia: implications for diagnosis and treatment." *International Review of Psychiatry*, 18(2), 95-107.

[118] Tang, Y. Y., et al. (2007). "Short-term meditation training improves attention and self-regulation." *Proceedings of the National Academy of Sciences*, 104(43), 17152-17156.

[119] Rao, T. S., et al. (2011). "Understanding nutrition, depression and mental illnesses." *Indian Journal of Psychiatry*, 53(2), 119-127.

[120] Homberg, J. R., & Lesch, K. P. (2011). "Looking on the bright side of serotonin transporter gene variation." *Biological Psychiatry*, 69(6), 513-519.

[121] Lovallo, W. R., et al. (2005). "Caffeine effects on cortisol secretion in men and women." *Psychoneuroendocrinology*, 30(4), 393-396.

[122] Ludwig, D. S. (2002). "The glycemic index: physiological mechanisms relating to obesity, diabetes, and cardiovascular disease." *JAMA*, 287(18), 2414-2423.

[123] Nishida, C., & Martinez, N. (Eds.). (2004). "Joint WHO/FAO Expert Consultation on Diet, Nutrition and the Prevention of Chronic Diseases." *Public Health Nutrition*, 7(1A), 245-250.

[124] Pasiakos, S. M., et al. (2015). "Protein requirements and optimal intakes in aging: Ample evidence supports elevated

protein intake for healthy aging." *Applied Physiology, Nutrition, and Metabolism*, 40(7), 684-689.

[125] Simopoulos, A. P. (2002). "The importance of the ratio of omega-6/omega-3 essential fatty acids." *Biomedicine & Pharmacotherapy*, 56(8), 365-379.

[126] Ludwig, D. S. (2002). "The glycemic index: physiological mechanisms relating to obesity, diabetes, and cardiovascular disease." *JAMA*, 287(18), 2414-2423.

[127] Young, S. N. (2007). "Folate and depression—a neglected problem." *Journal of Psychiatry and Neuroscience*, 32(2), 80-82.

[128] Brody, S., & Preut, R. (2002). "High-dose ascorbic acid increases intercourse frequency and improves mood: a randomized controlled clinical trial." *Biological Psychiatry*, 52(4), 371-374.

[129] de Baaij, J. H., et al. (2015). "Magnesium in man: implications for health and disease." *Physiological Reviews*, 95(1), 1-46.

[130] Smith, K. J., et al. (2018). "The therapeutic effects of adaptogens in fatigue, sleep, and depressive disorders." *CNS Drugs*, 32(1), 33-43.

[131] Eschenauer, G., & Sweet, B. V. (2006). "Pharmacology and therapeutic uses of theanine." *American Journal of Health-System Pharmacy*, 63(1), 26-30.

[132] Jakubowicz, D., et al. (2013). "High caloric intake at breakfast vs. dinner differentially influences weight loss of overweight and obese women." *Obesity*, 21(12), 2504-2512.

[133] Chandrasekhar, K., et al. (2012). "A prospective, randomized double-blind, placebo-controlled study of safety and efficacy of a high-concentration full-spectrum extract of ashwagandha root in reducing stress and anxiety in adults." *Indian Journal of Psychological Medicine*, 34(3), 255-262.

[134] Monteleone, P., et al. (1992). "Blunting by chronic phosphatidylserine administration of the stress-induced activation of the hypothalamo-pituitary-adrenal axis in healthy men." *European Journal of Clinical Pharmacology*, 42(4), 385-388.

[135] Nathan, P. J., et al. (2006). "The neuropharmacology of L-theanine (N-ethyl-L-glutamine): a possible neuroprotective and cognitive enhancing agent." *Journal of Herbal Pharmacotherapy*, 6(2), 21-30.

[136] Edwards, D., et al. (2012). "The effectiveness of Rhodiola rosea L. extract in reducing self-reported anxiety, stress, cognition, and other mood symptoms." *Phytotherapy Research*, 26(8), 1223-1229.

[137] Hill, E. E., et al. (2008). "Exercise and circulating cortisol levels: the intensity threshold effect." *Journal of Endocrinological Investigation*, 31(7), 587-591.

[138] Hamer, M. (2012). "Psychosocial stress and cardiovascular disease risk: the role of physical activity." *Psychosomatic Medicine*, 74(9), 896-903.

[139] Westcott, W. L. (2012). "Resistance training is medicine: effects of strength training on health." *Current Sports Medicine Reports*, 11(4), 209-216.

[140] Streeter, C. C., et al. (2010). "Effects of yoga versus walking on mood, anxiety, and brain GABA levels: a randomized controlled MRS study." *Journal of Alternative and Complementary Medicine*, 16(11), 1145-1152.

[141] Pascoe, M. C., et al. (2017). "Yoga, mindfulness-based stress reduction and stress-related physiological measures: A meta-analysis". *Psychoneuroendocrinology*, 86, 152-168.

[142] MacKenzie, B., & Maxwell, L. (2016). "Active recovery strategies and handover fatigue: A within-subjects pilot study comparing physical and cognitive stressors." *PLOS One*, 11(4), e0154536.

[143] Pedersen, B. K., & Hoffman-Goetz, L. (2000). "Exercise and the immune system: regulation, integration, and adaptation." *Physiological Reviews*, 80(3), 1055-1081.

[144] Calder, P. C., & Yaqoob, P. (2013). "Dietary manipulation of inflammation." *Proceedings of the Nutrition Society*, 72(3), 345-355.

[145] Maughan, R. J., et al. (2004). "Dietary supplements." *Journal of Sports Sciences*, 22(1), 95-113.

[146] Maintz, L., & Novak, N. (2007). "Histamine and histamine intolerance." *American Journal of Clinical Nutrition*, 85(5), 1185-1196.

[147] Girard, B., et al. (2007). "Human histamine N-methyltransferase gene (HNMT): chromosomal localization and tissue-specific expression." *Genomics*, 41(1), 115-120.

[148] Schwelberger, H. G. (2010). "Histamine intolerance: a metabolic disease?" *Inflammation Research*, 59, 219-221.

[149] Pascoe, M. C., et al. (2015). "Exercise and inflammatory responses to stressors: implications for immunological priming." *Journal of Physiology*, 593(24), 5279-5292.

[150] Comas-Basté, O., et al. (2019). "Histamine intolerance: the current state of the art." *Biomolecules*, 10(1), 118.

[151] Izzo, A. A., & Ernst, E. (2009). "Interactions between herbal medicines and prescribed drugs: a systematic review." *Drugs*, 61(15), 2163-2175.

[152] Hackney, A. C. (2006). "Stress and the neuroendocrine system: the role of exercise as a stressor and modifier of stress." *Expert Review of Endocrinology & Metabolism*, 1(6), 783-792.

[153] Schwingshackl, L., et al. (2018). "Dietary interventions to modulate chronic low-grade inflammation in metabolic syndrome: a systematic review and meta-analysis." *American Journal of Clinical Nutrition*, 107(4), 463-476.

[154] Kumar, S., & Babu, P. (2015). "Skin aging: a review of the process and its impact on daily life." *South Asian Journal of Cancer*, 4(3), 94-98.

[155] Jung, S. H., et al. (2014). "Irregular meal timing is associated with abdominal obesity and increased risk markers in healthy adults." *International Journal of Obesity*, 38(5), 526-532.

[156] Tremblay, F., & Marette, A. (2001). "Amino acid and insulin signaling via the mTOR/p70 S6 kinase pathway." *Journal of Biological Chemistry*, 276(38), 35574-35580.

[157] Calder, P. C. (2006). "Omega-3 polyunsaturated fatty acids and inflammation." *American Journal of Clinical Nutrition*, 83(6 Suppl), 1505S-1519S.

[158] Jenkins, D. J., et al. (2002). "Glycemic index: overview of implications in health and disease." *American Journal of Clinical Nutrition*, 76(1), 266S-273S.

[159] Clevers, H., & Bevins, C. L. (2013). "Paneth cells: maestros of the small intestinal crypts." *Annual Review of Physiology*, 75, 289-311.

[160] Boots, A. W., et al. (2008). "Quercetin as a potential anti-cancer agent: mechanisms of action and perspectives for future clinical use." *Biochemical Pharmacology*, 75(11), 1854-1863.

[161] Boots, A. W., et al. (2008). "Quercetin as a potential anti-cancer agent: mechanisms of action and perspectives for future clinical use." *Biochemical Pharmacology*, 75(11), 1854-1863.

[162] Randall, C., et al. (2008). "Randomized controlled trial of nettle sting for treatment of base-of-thumb pain." *Journal of the Royal Society of Medicine*, 101(2), 92-96.

[163] Brien, S., et al. (2004). "Systematic review of the use of bromelain in treatment of moderate and severe osteoarthritis." *BMJ Open*, 4(6), e005954.

[164] Eby, G. A., & Eby, K. L. (2006). "Rapid recovery from major depression using magnesium treatment." *Medical Hypotheses*, 67(2), 362-370.

[165] Johnston, C. S., & Huang, S. N. (1991). "Effect of ascorbic acid nutriture on blood histamine and neutrophil chemotaxis in guinea pigs." *Journal of Nutrition*, 121(1), 126-130.

[166] Johnston, C. S., & Huang, S. N. (1991). "Effect of ascorbic acid nutriture on blood histamine and neutrophil chemotaxis in guinea pigs." *Journal of Nutrition*, 121(1), 126-130.

[167] Nieman, D. C., et al. (2003). "Immune response to heavy exertion." *Journal of Applied Physiology*, 82(5), 1385-1394.

[168] Warburton, D. E., et al. (2006). "Health benefits of physical activity: the evidence." *Canadian Medical Association Journal*, 174(6), 801-809.

[169] Phillips, S. M., et al. (2012). "Resistance training in the older adult population: position statement from the national strength and conditioning association." *Journal of Strength and Conditioning Research*, 26(3), 543-580.

[170] Field, T. (2011). "Yoga clinical research review." *Complementary Therapies in Clinical Practice*, 17(1), 1-8.

[171] Barnes, J. N. (2015). "Exercise, cognitive function, and aging." *Advances in Physiology Education*, 39(2), 55-62.

[172] Wilding, J. P., et al. (2021). "Once-weekly semaglutide in adults with overweight or obesity." *New England Journal of Medicine*, 384(11), 989-1002.

[173] Smits, M. M., & Van Raalte, D. H. (2021). "Safety of semaglutide." *Frontiers in Endocrinology*, 12, 645563.

[174] Maughan, R. J., et al. (2004). "Dietary supplements." *Journal of Sports Sciences*, 22(1), 95-113.

[175] Lyssenko, V., et al. (2007). "Genetic variation in the GIPR locus is associated with impaired glucose and insulin responses in patients with type 2 diabetes." *Diabetologia*, 50(7), 1262-1270.

[176] Smits, M. M., & Van Raalte, D. H. (2021). "Safety of semaglutide." *Frontiers in Endocrinology*, 12, 645563.

[177] Hackney, A. C. (2006). "Stress and the neuroendocrine system: the role of exercise as a stressor and modifier of stress." *Expert Review of Endocrinology & Metabolism*, 1(6), 783-792.6

[178] Barclay, A. W., et al. (2008). "Glycemic index, glycemic load, and chronic disease risk—a meta-analysis of observational studies." *American Journal of Clinical Nutrition*, 87(3), 627-637.

[179] Erion, D. M., & Corkey, B. E. (2017). "Hyperinsulinemia: a cause of obesity?" *Current Obesity Reports*, 6(2), 178-186.

[180] Hackney, A. C. (2006). "Stress and the neuroendocrine system: the role of exercise as a stressor and modifier of stress." *Expert Review of Endocrinology & Metabolism*, 1(6), 783-792.

[181] Hackney, A. C. (2006). "Stress and the neuroendocrine system: the role of exercise as a stressor and modifier of stress." *Expert Review of Endocrinology & Metabolism*, 1(6), 783-792.

[182] Erion, D. M., & Corkey, B. E. (2017). "Hyperinsulinemia: a cause of obesity?" *Current Obesity Reports*, 6(2), 178-186.

[183] Layman, D. K., et al. (2003). "Increased dietary protein modifies glucose and insulin homeostasis in adult women during weight loss." *Journal of Nutrition*, 133(2), 405-410.

[184] Ros, E. (2010). "Health benefits of nut consumption." *Nutrients*, 2(7), 652-682.

[185] Gloyn, A. L., et al. (2003). "Large-scale association studies of variants in genes encoding the pancreatic beta-cell KATP channel subunits Kir6.2 (KCNJ11) and SUR1 (ABCC8)." *Diabetes*, 52(2), 568-572.

[186] Erion, D. M., & Corkey, B. E. (2017). "Hyperinsulinemia: a cause of obesity?" *Current Obesity Reports*, 6(2), 178-186.

[187] Jakubowicz, D., et al. (2013). "High caloric intake at breakfast vs. dinner differentially influences weight loss of overweight and obese women." *Obesity*, 21(12), 2504-2512.

[188] Yin, J., et al. (2008). "Efficacy of berberine in patients with type 2 diabetes mellitus." *Metabolism*, 57(5), 712-717.

[189] Khan, A., et al. (2003). "Cinnamon improves glucose and lipids of people with type 2 diabetes." *Diabetes Care*, 26(12), 3215-3218.

[190] Van Raalte, D. H., & Diamant, M. (2014). "Role of ZnT8 in insulin secretion and diabetes susceptibility." *Diabetologia*, 57(5), 883–886.

[191] Anderson, R. A., Broadhurst, C. L., Polansky, M. M., Schmidt, W. F., Khan, A., Flanagan, V. P., Schoene, N. W., & Graves, D. J. (2015). "Cinnamon improves glucose and lipids of people with type 2 diabetes." *Nutrition Journal*, 9, 43.

[192] Grant, S. F., Thorleifsson, G., Reynisdottir, I., Benediktsson, R., Manolescu, A., Sainz, J., & Stefansson, K. (2013). "TCF7L2 variant and risk of type 2 diabetes." *Diabetes*, 56(3), 879–882.

[193] Kahn, S. E., Hull, R. L., & Utzschneider, K. M. (2012). "Mechanisms linking obesity to insulin resistance and type 2 diabetes." *Nature*, 444(7121), 840–846.

[194] Anderson, R. A., et al. (1997). "Chromium picolinate improves glucose control in patients with type 2 diabetes: a randomized, double-blind, placebo-controlled trial." *Diabetes Care*, 20(4), 524-530.

[195] Jacob, S., et al. (1999). "Oral administration of RAC-alpha-lipoic acid modulates insulin sensitivity in patients with type-2 diabetes mellitus: a placebo-controlled pilot trial." *Free Radical Biology and Medicine*, 27(3-4), 309-314.

[196] Hackney, A. C. (2006). "Stress and the neuroendocrine system: the role of exercise as a stressor and modifier of stress." *Expert Review of Endocrinology & Metabolism*, 1(6), 783-792.

[197] Irvine, C., et al. (2018). "Resistance training improves glycemic control in obese type 2 diabetic men." *International Journal of Sports Medicine*, 39(06), 439-444.

[198] Gillen, J. B., & Gibala, M. J. (2014). "Is high-intensity interval training a time-efficient exercise strategy to improve health and fitness?" *Applied Physiology, Nutrition, and Metabolism*, 39(3), 409-412.

[199] Hawley, J. A., & Lessard, S. J. (2008). "Exercise training-induced improvements in insulin action." *Acta Physiologica*, 192(1), 127-135.

[200] Hawley, J. A., & Lessard, S. J. (2008). "Exercise training-induced improvements in insulin action." *Acta Physiologica*, 192(1), 127-135.

[201] Lee, S., et al. (2013). "Effects of exercise modality on insulin resistance and functional limitation in older adults: a randomized controlled trial." *Journal of Gerontology*, 68(2), 155-162.

[202] Black, D. S., & Slavich, G. M. (2016). "Mindfulness meditation and the immune system: a systematic review of randomized controlled trials." *Annals of the New York Academy of Sciences*, 1373(1), 13-24.

[203] Fisher, G., et al. (2018). "Mental stress and the metabolic syndrome: the role of adipose tissue cortisol reactivity." *Obesity*, 26(4), 770-776

[204] Jacob, S., et al. (1999). "Oral administration of RAC-alpha-lipoic acid modulates insulin sensitivity in patients with type-2 diabetes mellitus: a placebo-controlled pilot trial." *Free Radical Biology and Medicine*, 27(3-4), 309-314.

[205] Hutchison, E. R., et al. (2010). "Estrogen receptor-mediated regulation of microRNA inhibits let-7a expression and promotes cell proliferation in breast cancer." *Molecular Endocrinology*, 24(8), 1579-1590.

[206] Simpson, E. R., & Davis, S. R. (2001). "Minireview: Aromatase and the regulation of estrogen biosynthesis—some new perspectives." *Endocrinology*, 142(11), 4589-4594.

[207] Rossouw, J. E., et al. (2002). "Risks and benefits of estrogen plus progestin in healthy postmenopausal women: principal results: from the Women's Health Initiative randomized controlled trial." *JAMA*, 288(3), 321-333.

[208] Messina, M. (2014). "Soy foods, isoflavones, and the health of postmenopausal women." *The American Journal of Clinical Nutrition*, 100(Suppl_1), 423S-430S.

[209] Monteleone, P., et al. (1992). "Blunting by chronic phosphatidylserine administration of the stress-induced activation of the hypothalamo-pituitary-adrenal axis in healthy men." *European Journal of Clinical Pharmacology*, 42(4), 385-388.

[210] Mason, P., & Muller, C. (2014). "Vitamin and mineral supplements: what clinicians need to know." *Drugs & Therapy Perspectives*, 30(1), 12-17.

[211] Messina, M. (2014). "Soy foods, isoflavones, and the health of postmenopausal women." *The American Journal of Clinical Nutrition*, 100(Suppl_1), 423S-430S.

[212] Gamble, K. L., et al. (2014). "Shift work in nurses: contribution of phenotypes and genotypes to adaptation." *PLOS ONE*, 9(11), e112647.

[213] Hill, B. R., et al. (2021). "Severe caloric restriction reduces lean body mass but not preferentially over fat-free mass: a systematic review and meta-analysis." *Obesity Reviews*, 22(4), e13153.

[214] Hackney, A. C. (2006). "Stress and the neuroendocrine system: the role of exercise as a stressor and modifier of stress." *Expert Review of Endocrinology & Metabolism*, 1(6), 783-792.

[215] Hackney, A. C. (2006). "Stress and the neuroendocrine system: the role of exercise as a stressor and modifier of stress." *Expert Review of Endocrinology & Metabolism*, 1(6), 783-792.

[216] Nelson, H. D., et al. (2012). "Menopause and menopause symptoms." *Archives of Internal Medicine*, 172(5), 402-410.

[217] Simpson, E. R., & Davis, S. R. (2001). "Minireview: Aromatase and the regulation of estrogen biosynthesis—some new perspectives." *Endocrinology*, 142(11), 4589-4594.

[218] Ros, E. (2010). "Health benefits of nut consumption." *Nutrients*, 2(7), 652-682.

[219] Hu, F. B. (2003). "Plant-based foods and prevention of cardiovascular disease: an overview." *The American Journal of Clinical Nutrition*, 78(3 Suppl), 544S-551S.

[220] Monteleone, P., et al. (1992). "Blunting by chronic phosphatidylserine administration of the stress-induced activation of the hypothalamo-pituitary-adrenal axis in healthy men." *European Journal of Clinical Pharmacology*, 42(4), 385-388.

[221] Mason, P., & Muller, C. (2014). "Vitamin and mineral supplements: what clinicians need to know." *Drugs & Therapy Perspectives*, 30(1), 12-17

[222] Jarry, H., et al. (2010). "Role of ERβ in the effects of ERr 731 on the climacteric syndrome and bone." *Maturitas*, 65(3), 273-279.

[223] Heger-Mahn, D., et al. (2006). "The non-estrogenic alternative for the treatment of menopausal complaints: An overview of double-blind, placebo-controlled, randomized trials with ERr 731." *Maturitas*, 55, S30.

[224] Briot, K., & Roux, C. (2015). "Menopause and bone resorption." *Joint Bone Spine*, 82(5), 320-323.

[225] Tarleton, E. K., & Littenberg, B. (2015). "Magnesium intake and depression in adults." *Journal of the American Board of Family Medicine*, 28(2), 249-256.

[226] Hvas, A. M., & Nexo, E. (2006). "Diagnosis and treatment of vitamin B12 deficiency—an update." *Haematologica*, 91(11), 1506-1512

[227] Hackney, A. C. (2006). "Stress and the neuroendocrine system: the role of exercise as a stressor and modifier of stress." *Expert Review of Endocrinology & Metabolism*, 1(6), 783-792

[228] Sipilä, S., & Finni, T. (2016). "Physical activity and skeletal muscle adaptation during menopause." *Physical Activity and the Aging Brain*, Springer, 37-54.

[229] Pascoe, M. C., et al. (2017). "Yoga, mindfulness-based stress reduction and stress-related physiological measures: A meta-analysis." *Psychoneuroendocrinology*, 86, 152-168.

[230] Zhou, S. F., et al. (2009). "Polymorphism of human cytochrome P450 enzymes and its clinical impact." *Drug Metabolism Reviews*, 41(2), 89-295.

[231] Hayes, J. D., & Strange, R. C. (2000). "Glutathione S-transferase polymorphisms and their biological consequences." *Pharmacology*, 61(3), 154-166.

[232] Hein, D. W. (2009). "Molecular genetics and function of NAT1 and NAT2: role in aromatic amine metabolism and carcinogenesis." *Mutation Research*, 682(1), 13-23.

[233] Liska, D. (1998). "The detoxification enzyme systems." *Alternative Medicine Review*, 3(3), 187-198.

[234] Klein, A. V., & Kiat, H. (2015). "Detox diets for toxin elimination and weight management: a critical review of the evidence." *Journal of Human Nutrition and Dietetics*, 28(6), 675-686.

[235] Bailey, R. L., et al. (2011). "Why US adults use dietary supplements." *JAMA Internal Medicine*, 171(5), 355-359.

[236] Ginsberg, G., & Guyton, K. Z. (2009). "Genetic polymorphism in metabolism and host defense enzymes: implications for human health risk assessment." *Critical Reviews in Toxicology*, 39(7), 569-632.

[237] Zhou, S. F., et al. (2009). "Polymorphism of human cytochrome P450 enzymes and its clinical impact." *Drug Metabolism Reviews*, 41(2), 89-295.

[238] Blumberg, B., et al. (2011). "Obesogens: an emerging threat to public health." *American Journal of Obstetrics and Gynecology*, 202(5), 366-371.

[239] Epel, E. S., et al. (2000). "Stress may add bite to appetite in women: a laboratory study of stress-induced cortisol and eating behavior." *Psychoneuroendocrinology*, 26(1), 37-49.

[240] Zhou, S. F., et al. (2009). "Polymorphism of human cytochrome P450 enzymes and its clinical impact." *Drug Metabolism Reviews*, 41(2), 89-295.

[241] Lu, S. C. (2013). "Glutathione synthesis." *Biochimica et Biophysica Acta (BBA) - General Subjects*, 1830(5), 3143-3153.

[242] Ginsberg, G., & Guyton, K. Z. (2009). "Genetic polymorphism in metabolism and host defense enzymes: implications for human health risk assessment." *Critical Reviews in Toxicology*, 39(7), 569-632.

[243] Hayes, J. D., & Strange, R. C. (2000). "Glutathione S-transferase polymorphisms and their biological consequences." *Pharmacology*, 61(3), 154-166.

[244] Mason, P., & Muller, C. (2014). "Vitamin and mineral supplements: what clinicians need to know." *Drugs & Therapy Perspectives*, 30(1), 12-17.

[245] Anderson, R. A., & Kahlon, T. S. (2015). "Whole grains and blood lipid changes in apparently healthy adults: a systematic review and meta-analysis of randomized controlled trials." *Journal of Nutritional Science*, 4, e28.

[246] Cannon, B., & Nedergaard, J. (2004). "Brown adipose tissue: function and physiological significance." *Physiological Reviews*, 84(1), 277-359.

[247] Verhoeven, D. T., et al. (1997). "Epidemiological studies on brassica vegetables and cancer risk." *Cancer Epidemiology, Biomarkers & Prevention*, 6(9), 733-748.

[248] Jones, D. P. (2006). "Redox sensing: orthogonal control in cell cycle and apoptosis signaling." *Journal of Internal Medicine*, 268(5), 432-448.

[249] Packer, L., et al. (2005). "Antioxidant activity and biologic properties of a procyanidin-rich extract from pine (Pinus maritima) bark, Pycnogenol." *Free Radical Biology and Medicine,* 27(5-6), 704-724.

[250] Anderson, J. W., et al. (2009). "Health benefits of dietary fiber." *Nutrition Reviews,* 67(4), 188-205.

[251] Kaur, A., et al. (2008). "Effect of lemon peel extract on hepatic glutathione S-transferase activity in mice." *Pharmaceutical Biology,* 46(12), 854-858.

[252] Atkuri, K. R., et al. (2007). "N-Acetylcysteine—a safe antidote for cysteine/glutathione deficiency." *Current Opinion in Pharmacology,* 7(4), 355-359.

[253] Lu, S. C. (2013). "Glutathione synthesis." *Biochimica et Biophysica Acta (BBA) - General Subjects,* 1830(5), 3143-3153.

[254] Packer, L., et al. (1995). "Alpha-lipoic acid as a biological antioxidant." *Free Radical Biology and Medicine,* 19(2), 227-250.

[255] Anderson, J. W., et al. (2009). *Health benefits of dietary fiber. Nutrition Reviews,* 67(4), 188-205.

[256] Kennedy, D. O. (2016). "B Vitamins and the brain: mechanisms, dose and efficacy—a review." *Nutrients,* 8(2), 68.

[257] Ames, B. N. (2004). "Aging and mitochondrial decay: can mitochondrial DNA damage be reversed?" *Annals of the New York Academy of Sciences,* 1019(1), 221-225.

[258] Jones, D. P. (2006). "Redox sensing: orthogonal control in cell cycle and apoptosis signalling." *Journal of Internal Medicine,* 268(5), 432-448.

[259] Saller, R., et al. (2001). "The use of silymarin in the treatment of liver diseases." *Drugs,* 61(14), 2035-2063.

[260] Gebhardt, R. (1998). "Inhibition of cholesterol biosynthesis in primary cultured rat hepatocytes by artichoke (Cynara scolymus L.) extracts." *Journal of Pharmacology and Experimental Therapeutics,* 286(3), 1122-1128.

[261] Sharma, R. A., et al. (2005). "Pharmacodynamic and pharmacokinetic study of oral Curcuma extract in patients with colorectal cancer." *Clinical Cancer Research,* 11(20), 7485-7492.

[262] Ginsberg, G., & Guyton, K. Z. (2009). "Genetic polymorphism in metabolism and host defense enzymes: implications for human health risk assessment." *Critical Reviews in Toxicology*, 39(7), 569-632.

[263] Zhou, S. F., et al. (2009). "Polymorphism of human cytochrome P450 enzymes and its clinical impact." *Drug Metabolism Reviews*, 41(2), 89-295.

[264] Liska, D. (1998). "The detoxification enzyme systems." *Alternative Medicine Review*, 3(3), 187-198.

[265] Klein, A. V., & Kiat, H. (2015). Detox diets for toxin elimination and weight management: a critical review of the evidence. *Journal of Human Nutrition and Dietetics*, 28(6), 675-686.

[266] Mason, P., & Muller, C. (2014). "Vitamin and mineral supplements: what clinicians need to know." *Drugs & Therapy Perspectives*, 30(1), 12-17.

[267] Atkuri, K. R., et al. (2007). "N-Acetylcysteine—a safe antidote *Pharmacology*, 7(4), 355-359.

[268] Hackney, A. C. (2006). "Stress and the neuroendocrine system: the role of exercise as a stressor and modifier of stress." *Expert Review of Endocrinology & Metabolism*, 1(6), 783-792.

[269] Leicht, A. S., et al. (2003). "The effect of active versus passive recovery on cardiovascular function during the immediate post-exercise period." *Journal of Sports Sciences*, 21(1), 47-54.

[270] Ross, A., & Thomas, S. (2010). "The health benefits of yoga and exercise: a review of comparison studies." *Journal of Alternative and Complementary Medicine*, 16(1), 3-12.

[271] Beck, L. (1985). "The effect of rebounding on the immune system." *Journal of Applied Physiology*, 58(5), 1667.

[272] Irish, L. A., et al. (2015). "The role of sleep hygiene in promoting public health: a review of empirical evidence." *Sleep Medicine Reviews*, 22, 23-36.

[273] Walker, M. P. (2009). "The role of sleep in cognition and emotion." *Annals of the New York Academy of Sciences*, 1156(1), 168-197.

[274] Pascoe, M. C., et al. (2017). "Yoga, mindfulness-based stress reduction and stress-related physiological measures: A meta-analysis." *Psychoneuroendocrinology*, 86, 152-168.

[275] Chandola, T., et al. (2010). "Work stress and coronary heart disease: what are the mechanisms?" *European Heart Journal*, 31(5), 860-869.

[276] Turner, R., et al. (2021). *Genetics of Metabolic Diseases: Cholesterol and Cardiovascular Risks*. Oxford University Press.

[277] Rigat, B., et al. (1990). "An insertion/deletion polymorphism in the angiotensin I-converting enzyme gene accounting for half the variance of serum enzyme levels." *Journal of Clinical Investigation*, 86(4), 1343-1346.

[278] Nordestgaard, B. G., et al. (2010). "Lipoprotein(a) as a cardiovascular risk factor: present status." *Atherosclerosis*, 211(1), 41-44.

[279] Eichner, J. E., et al. (2002). "Apolipoprotein E polymorphism and cardiovascular disease: a huge review." *American Journal of Epidemiology*, 155(6), 487-495.

[280] Hackney, A. C. (2006). "Stress and the neuroendocrine system: the role of exercise as a stressor and modifier of stress." *Expert Review of Endocrinology & Metabolism*, 1(6), 783-792.

[281] Mason, P., & Muller, C. (2014). "Vitamin and mineral supplements: what clinicians need to know." *Drugs & Therapy Perspectives*, 30(1), 12-17.

[282] Chandola, T., et al. (2010). "Stress and coronary heart disease: what are the mechanisms?" *European Heart Journal*, 31(5), 860-869.

[283] Eichner, J. E., et al. (2002). "Apolipoprotein E polymorphism and cardiovascular disease: a huge review." *American Journal of Epidemiology*, 155(6), 487-495.

[284] Nordestgaard, B. G., et al. (2010). "Lipoprotein(a) as a cardiovascular risk factor: present status." *Atherosclerosis*, 211(1), 41-44.

[285] Rigat, B., et al. (1990). "An insertion/deletion polymorphism in the angiotensin I-converting enzyme gene

accounting for half the variance of serum enzyme levels." *Journal of Clinical Investigation*, 86(4), 1343-1346.

[286] Turner, R., et al. (2021). *Genetics of Metabolic Diseases: Cholesterol and Cardiovascular Risks.* Oxford University Press.

[287] Kris-Etherton, P. M., et al. (2002). "Omega-3 fatty acids in cardiovascular health." *Journal of Nutrition*, 132(3), 538-543.

[288] Kris-Etherton, P. M., et al. (2002). "Omega-3 fatty acids in cardiovascular health." *Journal of Nutrition*, 132(3), 538-543.

[289] Thompson, P. D., et al. (2003). "Exercise and cardiovascular disease prevention." *Circulation*, 107(24), e340-e346.

[290] Chandola, T., et al. (2010). "Stress and coronary heart disease: what are the mechanisms?" *European Heart Journal*, 31(5), 860-869.

[291] Anderson, J. W., et al. (2009). "Health benefits of dietary fiber." *Nutrition Reviews*, 67(4), 188-205.

[292] Appel, L. J., et al. (1997). "A clinical trial of the effects of dietary patterns on blood pressure." *New England Journal of Medicine*, 336(16), 1117-1124.

[293] He, F. J., & MacGregor, G. A. (2009). "A comprehensive review on salt and health and current experience of worldwide salt reduction programmes." *Journal of Human Hypertension*, 23(6), 363-384.

[294] Kris-Etherton, P. M., et al. (2002). "Omega-3 fatty acids in cardiovascular health." *Journal of Nutrition*, 132(3), 538-543.

[295] Kohlmeier, M. (2015). *Nutrient Metabolism: Omega-3s and Cardiovascular Health.* Academic Press.

[296] Mensink, R. P., et al. (2003). "Effects of dietary fatty acids and carbohydrates on the ratio of serum total to HDL cholesterol and on serum lipids and apolipoproteins: a meta-analysis of 60 controlled trials." *American Journal of Clinical Nutrition*, 77(5), 1146-1155.

[297] Burton-Freeman, B., & Sesso, H. D. (2010). "Antioxidants and cardiovascular disease: a review of clinical trials." *Current Atherosclerosis Reports*, 12(4), 244-250.

[298] Thompson, P. D., et al. (2003). "Exercise and cardiovascular disease prevention." *Circulation*, 107(24), e340-e346.

[299] Phillips, S. M., & Winett, R. A. (2010). "Uncomplicated resistance training and health-related outcomes: evidence for a public health mandate." *Current Sports Medicine Reports*, 9(4), 208-213.

[300] Nordestgaard, B. G., et al. (2010). "Lipoprotein(a) as a cardiovascular risk factor: present status." *Atherosclerosis*, 211(1), 41-44.

[301] Eichner, J. E., et al. (2002). "Apolipoprotein E polymorphism and cardiovascular disease: a huge review." *American Journal of Epidemiology*, 155(6), 487-495.

[302] Kris-Etherton, P. M., et al. (2002). "Omega-3 fatty acids in cardiovascular health." *Journal of Nutrition*, 132(3), 538-543.

[303] Hackney, A. C. (2006). "Stress and the neuroendocrine system: the role of exercise as a stressor and modifier of stress." *Expert Review of Endocrinology & Metabolism*, 1(6), 783-792.

[304] Mason, P., & Muller, C. (2014). "Vitamin and mineral supplements: what clinicians need to know." *Drugs & Therapy Perspectives*, 30(1), 12-17.

[305] Thompson, P. D., et al. (2003). "Exercise and cardiovascular disease prevention." *Circulation*, 107(24), e340-e346.

[306] Phillips, S. M., & Winett, R. A. (2010). "Uncomplicated resistance training and health-related outcomes: evidence for a public health mandate." *Current Sports Medicine Reports*, 9(4), 208-213.

[307] Sundell, J. (2011). "Resistance training is an effective tool against metabolic and frailty syndromes." *Advances in Preventive Medicine*, 2011, 984683.

[308] Chandola, T., et al. (2010). "Stress and coronary heart disease: what are the mechanisms?" *European Heart Journal*, 31(5), 860-869.

[309] Loos, R. J., et al. (2008). "The genetic predisposition for obesity and overeating: FTO and MC4R genes." *Nature Reviews Endocrinology*, 4(3), 189-197.

[310] Wardlaw, S. L. (2013). "Regulation of energy balance by the central nervous system: the role of MC4R." *Endocrinology and Metabolism Clinics*, 23(4), 725-739.

[311] Friedman, J. M., & Halaas, J. L. (1998). "Leptin and the regulation of body weight in mammals." *Nature*, 395(6704), 763-770.

[312] Cummings, D. E., & Overduin, J. (2007). "Ghrelin and the regulation of appetite." *Pharmacological Reviews*, 59(4), 424-438.

[313] Peters, J. C., et al. (2012). "Gene-diet interactions in the regulation of hunger and satiety." *Nutrition Reviews*, 70(12), 726-734.

[314] Tschöp, M., et al. (2000). "Circulating ghrelin levels are decreased in human obesity." *Diabetes*, 49(8), 1349-1352.

[315] Greenway, F. L., et al. (2009). "Appetite regulation by blood glucose and hormonal control." *Nutrition Reviews*, 67(10), 589-597.

[316] Cummings, D. E., & Overduin, J. (2007). "Ghrelin and the regulation of appetite." *Pharmacological Reviews*, 59(4), 424-438.

[317] Hebebrand, J., et al. (2010). "Weight loss strategies and genetic predisposition." *Obesity Facts*, 3(2), 105-117.

[318] Volkow, N. D., & Wise, R. A. (2005). "How can drug addiction help us understand obesity?" *Nature Neuroscience*, 8(5), 555-560.

[319] Jansen, A., et al. (2003). "Appetite suppressants and their effects on craving intensity." *Appetite*, 41(3), 291-298.

[320] Kristeller, J. L., & Wolever, R. Q. (2011). "Mindfulness-based eating awareness training for treating binge eating disorder: The conceptual foundation." *Eating Disorders*, 19(1), 49-61.

[321] Peters, J. C., et al. (2012). "Gene-diet interactions in the regulation of hunger and satiety." *Nutrition Reviews*, 70(12), 726-734.

[322] Klok, M. D., et al. (2007). "The role of leptin and ghrelin in the regulation of food intake and body weight in humans: a review." *Obesity Reviews*, 8(1), 21-34.

[323] Greenway, F. L., et al. (2009). "Appetite regulation by blood glucose and hormonal control." *Nutrition Reviews*, 67(10), 589-597.

[324] Hebebrand, J., et al. (2010). "Weight loss strategies and genetic predisposition." *Obesity Facts*, 3(2), 105-117.

[325] Sumithran, P., et al. (2011). "Long-term persistence of hormonal adaptations to weight loss." *New England Journal of Medicine*, 365(17), 1597-1604.

[326] Pereira, M. A., et al. (2004). "Fiber-rich diets and craving reduction." *Journal of Nutrition*, 134(3), 613-618.

[327] Pereira, M. A., et al. (2004). "Fiber-rich diets and craving reduction." *Journal of Nutrition*, 134(3), 613-618.

[328] Parra, D., et al. (2008). "Dietary conjugated linoleic acid and body composition." *Journal of Nutrition*, 138(6), 1128-1135.

[329] Brand-Miller, J. C., et al. (2002). "Dietary glycemic index: health implications." *Journal of the American College of Nutrition*, 21(6), 408-416.

[330] Hebebrand, J., et al. (2010). "Weight loss strategies and genetic predisposition." *Obesity Facts*, 3(2), 105-117.

[331] Hayamizu, K., et al. (2003). "Effect of garcinia cambogia extract on serum insulin and appetite." *International Journal of Obesity*, 27(5), 649-656.

[332] Cummings, D. E., & Overduin, J. (2007). "Ghrelin and the regulation of appetite." *Pharmacological Reviews*, 59(4), 424-438.

[333] Peters, J. C., et al. (2012). "Gene-diet interactions in the regulation of hunger and satiety." *Nutrition Reviews*, 70(12), 726-734.

[334] Tschöp, M., et al. (2000). "Circulating ghrelin levels are decreased in human obesity." *Diabetes*, 49(8), 1349-1352.

[335] Greenway, F. L., et al. (2009). "Appetite regulation by blood glucose and hormonal control." *Nutrition Reviews*, 67(10), 589-597.

[336] Cummings, D. E., & Overduin, J. (2007). "Ghrelin and the regulation of appetite." *Pharmacological Reviews*, 59(4), 424-438.

[337] Pereira, M. A., et al. (2004). "Fiber-rich diets and craving reduction." *Journal of Nutrition*, 134(3), 613-618.

[338] Epel, E. S., et al. (2001). "Stress may add bite to appetite in women: a laboratory study of stress-induced cortisol and eating behavior." *Psychoneuroendocrinology*, 26(1), 37-49.

[339] Pereira, M. A., et al. (2004). "Fiber-rich diets and craving reduction." *Journal of Nutrition*, 134(3), 613-618.

[340] Parra, D., et al. (2008). "Dietary conjugated linoleic acid and body composition." *Journal of Nutrition*, 138(6), 1128-1135.

[341] Chiesa, A., et al. (2013). "Mindfulness-based therapy for emotional eating and cravings: A systematic review." *Journal of Clinical Psychology*, 69(1), 28-44.

[342] Heck, A. M., et al. (2000). "Garcinia cambogia for weight loss." *Journal of the American Dietetic Association*, 100(10), 1158-1161.

[343] Rausch, P., et al. (2011). "A novel assay for the identification of FUT2 secretor status correlates with Crohn's disease susceptibility." *Human Mutation*, 32(9), 1000-1005.

[344] Tap, J., et al. (2009). "Towards the human intestinal microbiota phylogenetic core." *Environmental Microbiology*, 11(10), 2574-2584.

[345] Ingram, C. J., et al. (2009). "Lactose digestion and the evolutionary genetics of lactase persistence." *Human Genetics*, 124(6), 579-591.

[346] Misselwitz, B., et al. (2013). "Lactose malabsorption and intolerance: pathogenesis, diagnosis, and treatment." *United European Gastroenterology Journal*, 1(3), 151-159.

[347] Kühn, R., et al. (1993). "Interleukin-10-deficient mice develop chronic enterocolitis." *Cell*, 75(2), 263-274.

[348] Abraham, C., & Cho, J. H. (2009). "Inflammatory bowel disease." *New England Journal of Medicine*, 361(21), 2066-2078.

[349] Dale, H. F., et al. (2019). "The influence of a gluten-free diet on gut microbiota composition in healthy non-celiac individuals: a systematic review." *Clinical Nutrition*, 38(6), 2402-2410.

[350] Halmos, E. P., et al. (2015). "Diets that differ in their FODMAP content alter the colonic luminal microenvironment." *Gut*, 64(1), 93-100.

[351] Sanders, M. E., et al. (2013). "Probiotics and prebiotics in intestinal health and disease: from biology to the clinic." *Nature Reviews Gastroenterology & Hepatology*, 10(9), 605-614.

[352] Dale, H. F., et al. (2019). "The influence of a gluten-free diet on gut microbiota composition in healthy non-celiac individuals: a systematic review." *Clinical Nutrition*, 38(6), 2402-2410.

[353] Halmos, E. P., et al. (2015). "Diets that differ in their FODMAP content alter the colonic luminal microenvironment." *Gut*, 64(1), 93-100.

[354] Gibson, G. R., & Roberfroid, M. B. (1995). "Dietary modulation of the human colonic microbiota: introducing the concept of prebiotics." *Journal of Nutrition*, 125(6), 1401-1412.

[355] Martinsen, T. C., et al. (2005). "Regulation of gastric acid secretion." *Gut*, 54(1), 13-22.

[356] Calder, P. C. (2017). "Omega-3 fatty acids and inflammatory processes: from molecules to man." *Biochemical Society Transactions*, 45(5), 1105-1115.

[357] Misselwitz, B., et al. (2013). "Lactose malabsorption and intolerance: pathogenesis, diagnosis, and treatment." *United European Gastroenterology Journal*, 1(3), 151-159.

[358] Marco, M. L., et al. (2017). "Health benefits of fermented foods: microbiota and beyond." *Current Opinion in Biotechnology*, 44, 94-102.

[359] Martinsen, T. C., et al. (2005). "Regulation of gastric acid secretion." *Gut*, 54(1), 13-22.

[360] Sanders, M. E., et al. (2013). "Probiotics and prebiotics in intestinal health and disease: from biology to the clinic." *Nature Reviews Gastroenterology & Hepatology*, 10(9), 605-614.

[361] Kim, S. K., & Park, J. H. (2014). "Probiotic Lactobacillus paracasei enhances gut health and immune function." *Journal of Microbiology*, 52(5), 476-481.

[362] Yamano, T., et al. (2006). "Effect of Bifidobacterium bifidum Bb-02 on human gastrointestinal function." *Bioscience of Microbiota, Food and Health*, 25(2), 105-112.

[363] Szilagyi, A. (2002). "Lactose intolerance, dairy avoidance, and treatment options." *Nutrition in Clinical Practice*, 17(1), 84-89.

[364] de Vries, M. C., et al. (2006). "Lactobacillus plantarum— survival, functional and potential probiotic properties in the human intestinal tract." *International Dairy Journal*, 16(9), 1018-1028.

[365] Kalliomäki, M., et al. (2003). "Probiotics and the prevention of atopic disease: a randomized, placebo-controlled trial." *The Lancet*, 361(9372), 1869-1871.

[366] Mayer, E. A. (2011). "Gut feelings: the emerging biology of gut-brain communication." *Nature Reviews Neuroscience*, 12(8), 453-466.

[367] Monda, V., et al. (2017). "Exercise modifies the gut microbiota with positive health effects." *Oxidative Medicine and Cellular Longevity*, 2017, 3831972.

[368] Bordoni, B., et al. (2018). "The influence of breathing on the central nervous system." *Journal of Multidisciplinary Healthcare*, 11, 133-139

[369] Bordoni, B., et al. (2018). "The influence of breathing on the central nervous system." *Journal of Multidisciplinary Healthcare*, 11, 133-139

[370] Konturek, P. C., et al. (2011). "Stress and the gut: pathophysiology, clinical consequences, diagnostic approach and treatment options." *Journal of Physiology and Pharmacology*, 62(6), 591-599.

[371] Benedict, C., et al. (2016). "Gut microbiota and sleep." *Current Sleep Medicine Reports*, 2(2), 1-6.

[372] Popkin, B. M., et al. (2010). "Water, hydration, and health." *Nutrition Reviews*, 68(8), 439-458.

[373] Lehrke, M., & Lazar, M. A. (2005). "The many faces of PPARgamma." *Cell*, 123(6), 993-999.

[374] Robitaille, J., et al. (2003). "The PPARgamma P12A polymorphism modulates the relationship between dietary fat intake and components of the metabolic syndrome." *Clinical Genetics*, 63(2), 109-116.

[375] Large, V., et al. (1997). "Adrenergic regulation of lipolysis in human fat cells." *Journal of Lipid Research*, 38(6), 1155-1161.

[376] Meirhaeghe, A., et al. (2000). "Beta2-adrenoceptor gene polymorphism, body weight, and physical activity." *The Lancet*, 356(9246), 190-191.

[377] Baier, L. J., & Bogardus, C. (1999). "Genetic variation in the FABP2 gene and insulin resistance." *Journal of Clinical Investigation*, 103(1), 79-85.

[378] Carlsson, M., et al. (2000). "Fatty acid-binding protein-2 gene Thr54 mutation is associated with increased fat oxidation and insulin resistance." *Diabetes Care*, 23(2), 235-239.

[379] Thorens, B. (2015). "GLUT2, glucose sensing and glucose homeostasis." *Diabetes & Metabolism*, 41(2), 51-56.

[380] Guillam, M. T., et al. (1997). "Early diabetes and abnormal postnatal pancreatic islet development in mice lacking Glut-2." *Nature Genetics*, 17(3), 327-330.

[381] Hu, T., et al. (2012). "Effects of low-carbohydrate diets versus low-fat diets on metabolic risk factors." *American Journal of Epidemiology*, 176(suppl_7), S44-S54.

[382] Martin, C. K., et al. (2007). "Effect of calorie restriction on resting metabolic rate and spontaneous physical activity." *Obesity*, 15(12), 2964-2973.

[383] Jenkins, D. J., et al. (2001). "High-protein diets in hyperlipidemia." *American Journal of Clinical Nutrition*, 74(1), 57-63.

[384] Meirhaeghe, A., et al. (2000). "Beta2-adrenoceptor gene polymorphism, body weight, and physical activity." *The Lancet*, 356(9246), 190-191.

[385] Carlsson, M., et al. (2000). "Fatty acid-binding protein-2 gene Thr54 mutation is associated with increased fat oxidation and insulin resistance." *Diabetes Care*, 23(2), 235-239.

[386] Hu, T., et al. (2012). "Effects of low-carbohydrate diets versus low-fat diets on metabolic risk factors." *American Journal of Epidemiology*, 176(suppl_7), S44-S54.

[387] Jenkins, D. J., et al. (2001). "High-protein diets in hyperlipidemia." *American Journal of Clinical Nutrition*, 74(1), 57–63.

[388] Houweling, P. J., et al. (2018). "Is evolutionary loss our gain? The role of ACTN3 p.Arg577Ter (R577X) genotype in athletic performance, ageing, and disease." *Human Mutation*, 39(12), 1774–1787.

[389] Velloso, C. P. (2008). "Regulation of muscle mass by growth hormone and IGF-I." *British Journal of Pharmacology*, 154(3), 557–568.

[390] Rodgers, B. D., & Garikipati, D. K. (2008). "Clinical, agricultural, and evolutionary biology of myostatin: a comparative review." *Endocrine Reviews*, 29(5), 513–534.

[391] Schiaffino, S., & Reggiani, C. (2011). "Fiber types in mammalian skeletal muscles." *Physiological Reviews*, 91(4), 1447–1531.

[392] Gillen, J. B., & Gibala, M. J. (2014). "Is high-intensity interval training a time-efficient exercise strategy to improve health and fitness?" *Applied Physiology, Nutrition, and Metabolism*, 39(3), 409–412.

[393] Stokes, T., et al. (2018). "Recent perspectives regarding the role of dietary protein for the promotion of muscle hypertrophy with resistance exercise training." *Nutrients*, 10(2), 180.

[394] Houweling, P. J., et al. (2018). "Is evolutionary loss our gain? The role of ACTN3 p.Arg577Ter (R577X) genotype in athletic performance, ageing, and disease." *Human Mutation*, 39(12), 1774–1787.

[395] Velloso, C. P. (2008). "Regulation of muscle mass by growth hormone and IGF-I." *British Journal of Pharmacology*, 154(3), 557–568.

[396] Rodgers, B. D., & Garikipati, D. K. (2008). "Clinical, agricultural, and evolutionary biology of myostatin: a comparative review." *Endocrine Reviews*, 29(5), 513–534.

[397] Hawley, J. A., & Leckey, J. J. (2015). "Carbohydrate dependence during prolonged, intense endurance exercise." *Sports Medicine*, 45(Suppl 1), 5–12.

[398] Morton, R. W., et al. (2015). "Protein supplementation to augment resistance training-induced increases in muscle mass and strength." *Sports Medicine*, 45(1), 111–131.

[399] Jäger, R., et al. (2017). "International Society of Sports Nutrition position stand: protein and exercise." *Journal of the International Society of Sports Nutrition*, 14(1), 20.

[400] Thomas, D. T., et al. (2016). "Position of the Academy of Nutrition and Dietetics, Dietitians of Canada, and the American College of Sports Medicine: nutrition and athletic performance." *Journal of the Academy of Nutrition and Dietetics*, 116(3), 501–528.

[401] Tisdale, M. J. (2009). "Mechanisms of cancer cachexia." *Physiological Reviews*, 89(2), 381–410.

[402] Powers, S. K., et al. (2004). "Exercise-induced oxidative stress: cellular mechanisms and impact on muscle force production." *Physiological Reviews*, 94(2), 435–448.

[403] Santos, D. A., et al. (2014). "Magnesium intake is associated with strength performance in elite basketball, handball and volleyball players." *Magnesium Research*, 27(2), 61–69.

[404] Sawka, M. N., et al. (2007). "American College of Sports Medicine position stand. Exercise and fluid replacement." *Medicine & Science in Sports & Exercise*, 39(2), 377–390.

[405] Kennedy, D. O. (2016). "B Vitamins and the brain: mechanisms, dose and efficacy—a review." *Nutrients*, 8(2), 68.

[406] Miller, K. C., et al. (2010). "Electrolyte and plasma volume shifts in response to muscle cramp protocol." *Medicine & Science in Sports & Exercise*, 42(5), 953–961.

[407] Miller, K. C., et al. (2010). "Electrolyte and plasma volume shifts in response to muscle cramp protocol." *Medicine & Science in Sports & Exercise*, 42(5), 953–961.

[408] Peake, J. M. (2019). "Vitamin C: effects of exercise and requirements with training." *Nutrients*, 11(9), 1944.

[409] Kreher, J. B. (2016). "Diagnosis and prevention of overtraining syndrome: an opinion on education strategies." *Open Access Journal of Sports Medicine*, 7, 115–122.

[410] Kraemer, W. J., & Ratamess, N. A. (2004). "Fundamentals of resistance training: progression and exercise prescription." *Medicine & Science in Sports & Exercise*, 36(4), 674–688.

[411] Bevan, H. R., et al. (2010). "Optimal loading for the development of peak power output in professional rugby players." *Journal of Strength and Conditioning Research*, 24(1), 43–47.

[412] Behm, D. G., & Chaouachi, A. (2011). "A review of the acute effects of static and dynamic stretching on performance." *European Journal of Applied Physiology*, 111(11), 2633–2651.

[413] Simpson, N. S., et al. (2017). "Sleep and human performance." *Current Opinion in Physiology*, 15, 123–129.

Made in United States
Cleveland, OH
23 April 2025

16363025R00184